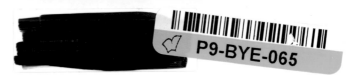

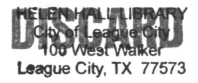

One Hundred Autobiographies

One Hundred Autobiographies

A Memoir

David Lehman

Cornell University Press

Ithaca and London

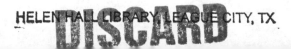

First published 2019 by Cornell University Press

Printed in the United States of America

Library of Congress Cataloging-in-Publication Data

Names: Lehman, David, 1948– author.
Title: One hundred autobiographies : a memoir / David Lehman.
Description: Ithaca [New York] : Cornell University Press, 2019.
Identifiers: LCCN 2019019614 (print) | LCCN 2019020574 (ebook) |
    ISBN 9781501746475 (epub/mobi) | ISBN 9781501746468 (pdf) |
    ISBN 9781501746451 | ISBN 9781501746451 (cloth)
Subjects: LCSH: Lehman, David, 1948– —Health. | Bladder—Cancer—Patients—
    Biography. | Poets, American—Biography.
Classification: LCC RC280.B5 (ebook) | LCC RC280.B5 L45 2019 (print) | DDC
    616.99/4620092 [B]—dc23
LC record available at https://lccn.loc.gov/2019019614

For Stacey

Contents

Preface   *xiii*

1 Execution Poem Expert   *1*

2 Spots of Time   *3*

3 Café Loup   *4*

4 No Big Deal   *6*

5 Cancer Alley   *9*

6 The Crisis   *10*

7 The Aftermath   *12*

8 The Procedure   *13*

9 The Protocol   *14*

10 The Good Kind   *16*

11 The Diarist   *18*

12 None But the Strong   *20*

13 Tropic of Cancer   *22*

14 Hospitals and Airports   *24*

15 Back to the Waiting Room   *26*

16 "Hurry up, please, it's time"   *28*

17 Why 1963?   *29*

18 Good Friday   *33*

19 *Lasciate ogni speranza, voi ch'entrate!*   *35*

20 The Weekend Before   *37*

21 "Bladder cancer: Isn't that what Sinatra died of?"   *39*

22 In a Technical Sense   *41*

23 Five O'Clock Rush   *42*

24 A Heart Event   *44*

25 Good Show   *46*

26 Metaport   *47*

27 If You Were an English Poet   *49*

28 The Regimen   *51*

29 A Few Beacons in the Quicksand   *53*

30 What's the Story?   *57*

31 Time Is on My Side   *59*

32 Rush Job   *63*

33 Final Call   *64*

34 And Then You Crash   *66*

35 Chemo   *68*

36 Roid Rage   *72*

37 Under the Garden   *74*

38 The End   *77*

39 Falling in Love Again   *78*

40 Nothingness   *80*

41 Syllabus   *81*

42 Commencement Speech   *84*

43 The Exquisite Corpse   *86*

44 The Editorial "We"   *87*

45 Oblivion   *89*

46 Dostoyevsky   *91*

47 The Spiritual Connection   *93*

48 "Myself, When Stoned"   *95*

49 Bloomsday   *98*

50 Tom Collins   *100*

51 The Admissions Officer   *102*

52 Columbia   *107*

53 Classic Koch   *111*

54 The Poem Team   *116*

55 Shakespeare's Birthday   *118*

56 Recovery Room   *121*

57 The Rebbe   *123*

58 Life Begins at Forty   *127*

59 Search for Meaning   *131*

60 The Old Religion   *133*

61 The Problem of Evil   *136*

62 Dean Martin's Hat   *137*

63 740 Francs   *139*

64 Shalom Aleichem Rides to the Rescue   *141*

65 The Arrival of the Messiah   *143*

66 Sabbath Services   *145*

67 A Complicated Guy   *148*

68 The Patient Next to You   *151*

69 Cambridge   *154*

70 Armistice Day, 1970   *156*

71 The Sublime Pain of Being   *158*

72 The Glass Skeleton   *160*

73 Why Does the Bridge Not Progress?   *163*

74 Q & A   *165*

75 Ludlowville, 1981   *169*

76 Bio Note (Alt.)   *171*

77 Wedding Ceremony   *174*

78 Moscow, 2007   *177*

79 Group Therapy   *180*

80 Fort Tryon Park   *181*

81 A Fine Invention   *182*

82 Identity Theft   *184*

83 A Routine Visit   *186*

84 Doctor Jew   *188*

85 "Except for the cancer ..."   *192*

86 The Heart Knows   *194*

87 A Black Dress   *195*

88 Heisenberg as Hero   *197*

89 Cheers!   *199*

90 Walter Lehmann   *200*

91 Rowing in Eden   *203*

92 I Remember Mama   *205*

93 No Regrets   *208*

94 If I Could   *212*

95 The Scar   *213*

96 The Secret   *214*

97 Like a Hurricane   *215*

98 In the Eyes of the Beholder   *217*

99 Champagne Cocktails   *219*

100 In the Swim   *221*

Preface

The title of this book, *One Hundred Autobiographies*, was a high-concept prompt in three words. It was Mark Strand's title. He said he hoped to get around to writing a book worthy of it. In 2014, when he was dying of one form of cancer while I was battling another, he said that I could have the title if he didn't get there first. Mark, a brilliant poet and dear friend, with whom I had collaborated on a number of projects, including *The Best American Poetry 1991*, died at the age of eighty on November 29, 2014.

One week after Mark's death, my heart stopped for a few seconds because something went wrong with the anesthesia following a bad news procedure at the hospital. Chemotherapy, a preferred modern term for the valley of the shadow of death, came next. During my descent into that lonesome valley, I found that writing every day, no matter how bad the pain, was one way I had to keep myself going. Writing was keeping me alive—more, it was asserting my will to live. And now, with the gift of Mark's title, I had a framework—and could craft a form—for the thoughts, dreams, memories, hopes, fears, and fantasies that occupied my mind as I entered the unknown territory from whose bound few travelers return.

As a patient, confined to bed or limited in your mobility, you have a lot of time to think. Some irrecoverable hours are spent watching cable news, athletic events, television shows, old movies. The need to escape is great, and the third or fourth time you see *The Wild Bunch* or *Double Indemnity* is time you won't regret. Still, these are passive activities. How much greater it is to create something out of the debris of one's consciousness—something that is itself a living thing—a book in a form all its own.

The ordeal that I endured as a cancer patient was not the only subject that engaged me. Battling a disease that may end your life, you quite naturally take stock—you think about where you've come from, what you've done and not done, whom you have loved, whether you've measured up to expectation, how you have affected the lives of others. In these circumstances a journal about the present can easily interrupt itself to accommodate a memory or a dream.

"Creative nonfiction" has acquired legitimacy as a literary category, and I benefited from the freedom to deviate from a strict orderly procession of fact. One model for what I was doing is the work of Machado de Assis, the great nineteenth-century Brazilian novelist, author of *Epitaph of a Small Winner* and *Dom Casmurro*, who wrote in short numbered sections that allowed him to digress at will. Machado joined the Byron of *Don Juan* as masters of the calculated interruption, who would elevate digression to an aesthetic ideal.

The idea of autobiographies, plural, had a further appeal to one who is attracted, as I am, to the idea of the heteronym as introduced and perfected by the Portuguese poet Fernando Pessoa. A heteronym goes the pseudonym one better: not only a false name but a distinctive style and a full biography go to all the authors Pessoa perpetuated. I flipped things a bit in *One Hundred Autobiographies* by assigning the same name to multiple personae and by switching from "I" to "you" to "he" as if the pronoun governed more than the point of view.

And I would mention a third influence: *The Singing Detective* by Dennis Potter, a series of six television episodes centering on a hospitalized writer with an active memory and a penchant for melodramatic fantasy. We go from memory to imagination, from one time zone to another, and, since the protagonist is a writer, we also enter the realm of the novel he is writing, if only in his mind. The protagonist has, except for the terminal "e" in Marlowe, the same name as Raymond Chandler's detective hero portrayed by Humphrey Bogart in *The Big Sleep* and Robert Mitchum in *Farewell, My Lovely*. Potter's Philip Marlow is three individuals in one damaged skin. The tuxedo-clad hard-boiled crooner of noir fiction and fantasy. The remembered ten-year-old lad in wartime England. The middle-aged man in the London hospital ward with an ex-wife he suspects is having an affair with a rival who may or may not exist.

To make matters even more happily complex, the characters are likely now and then to break into song, mouthing the words of tunes popular in 1945. You hear the voices of Bing Crosby and the Andrews Sisters ("Accentuate the Positive"), Al Jolson ("After You've Gone"), the Mills Brothers ("Paper Doll"). Each episode begins with an instrumental of "Peg o' My Heart" (Max Harris). Vera Lynn sings "We'll Meet Again" at series' end.

I, too, like to punctuate my memories with melodies. Not a day goes by without my listening to one or another great song, not a week without writing about a piece of music, as the other night I did when listening to Jerry Hadley and Frederica Von Stade sing "Make Believe" and "Why Do I Love You?"—as if writing about the experience would be enough to make it come to life in the reader's ear.

One Hundred Autobiographies has one central narrative within which other stories come and go. The "fake memoir" has gained credibility among writers in recent years, and it is only fair to warn the reader that facts sometimes dissolve into fiction in the writer's mind—usually when the truth requires it. Let me explain with an example. In Australia, home of great poetry hoaxes, the poet Gwen Harwood wrote poems under the pseudonym "Walter Lehmann" to expose the biases of a certain editor. The hoax took place in the early 1960s, and when I learned about it I felt like claiming Walter Lehmann as an uncle and treating him as such in the chapter devoted to him.

It has happened that people meeting me have assumed that I belong to the great Lehman family that has been notable in public service and philanthropy. It is possible that the frequency of this and similar errors were sources of inspiration when I went to the computer and wrote my five hundred words of the day.

But mostly what I set out to write was a portrait of my mind and what it made of the experience of life and death. I had excellent doctors, but the person who deserves the most credit for my survival is my wife, Stacey, to whom this book is lovingly and most gratefully dedicated.

—*September 16, 2018*

1

Execution Poem Expert

On June 11, 2001, CBS News in New York City called to see whether I, a poet and professor, would appear on a daytime news show to explain why Timothy McVeigh's last words took the form of W. E. Henley's "Invictus" (1875), an old warhorse of a poem, sixteen lines long, handwritten by the prisoner on death row and handed to the warden. McVeigh was facing the lethal injection because he had detonated the bomb that killed 168, wounding hundreds more, in Oklahoma City in 1995, in the single worst act of domestic terrorism in the nation's history.

McVeigh was convicted, he was condemned, but he wasn't ready to flinch. "Invictus" is Latin for "invincible," and McVeigh was presenting himself as defiant, proud: "My head is bloody, but unbowed." The poem's conclusion: "I am the master of my fate: / I am the captain of my soul." That the bomber would represent himself with a poem was noteworthy, and CBS needed someone with the literary credentials to talk about the choice and how it reflected the mind of a mass murderer facing execution.

It was my birthday, and the TV appearance was, as far as I was concerned, a lark, an adventure, or an auspicious omen. I went through the various stages that precede even a bit performance on television—the endless rehearsals of things you have told them

you would say, the application of makeup. The task was not oner-
ous. I knew just enough about Henley to locate him in the anchor-
person's mind, and the poem is straightforward enough. You could
tell what McVeigh meant to say.

The CBS producer, an efficient Wellesley alumna, was in a rush,
as the job required. But she took the time to ask me whether I pro-
nounce my name "Lee-man" or "Lay-man."

"Lee-man," I said.

As I sat in the greenroom waiting for my three-minute stint be-
fore the cameras, I watched the program. Heading for break, the
screen announced what was coming: "Execution Poem Expert."

What a wonderful distinction, I thought. My wife, Stacey, made
me business cards with these words on them.

And when I got on the air, I was introduced as David Lay-man.

That is what I mean by a spot of time.

2

Spots of Time

It was Wordsworth who introduced the phrase. In *The Prelude*, his autobiographical epic, Wordsworth wrote, "There are in our existence spots of time, / That with distinct pre-eminence retain / A renovating virtue," such that, in unhappy or humdrum circumstances, they leave our minds "nourished and invisibly repaired." A spot of time, recollected and stored in the memory, "enables us to mount, / When high, more high, and lifts us up when fallen."

This is a deservedly famous passage—or used to be, when English majors were many and all were required to read the major romantic poets. I would, however, insist that the moments and hours that transcend the here-and-now and make so lasting an impression are not limited to ones that gave pleasure the first time around. On the contrary, the recollection of a melancholy or painful episode—an emotional crisis, an illness, an accident, a humiliation, even the death of a loved one—may perform the "renovating virtue" that Wordsworth described. The memory may be involuntary, triggered by an uncanny sense of repetition, or provoked by the act of writing, as I hope to demonstrate here.

3

Café Loup

The Harvard professor's lecture on *The Prelude* was as brilliant as advertised. The professor linked the passage I just quoted to comparable instances of recollection and "renovating virtue" in Wordsworth's "Immortality Ode" and "I Wandered Lonely as a Cloud." When he quoted from memory the magnificent last paragraph of Ralph Waldo Emerson's great essay "Compensation," the audience was as moved as it was impressed. I moderated the lively question-and-answer session that followed, which went off without a hitch, and the students lined up to get their books signed by the distinguished lecturer. It was a perk of the job that I got to take the professor out to dinner and drinks to cap off the evening in celebratory fashion, and we went to Café Loup, the bar on Thirteenth Street west of Sixth Avenue where the food is lousy but the pour is generous. We arrived in good cheer but, to my astonishment, our guest, so erudite and knowledgeable in the lecture hall, was, when relaxed, an old-fashioned bore: someone who talks your head off without pause. From the first taste of his single-malt scotch on the rocks, my guest talked, and talked, and talked. Now he was holding forth to a captive audience of three of my colleagues, a graduate student, and my wife about China's theft of our intellectual property while the listeners sipped their cocktails and fidgeted with their napkins. I motioned to the waiter ("another round for everyone") and excused myself to the men's room. But instead of finding refuge, I glanced down to see that I had pissed blood in the icy white urinal. It was ugly, like cracking an egg to find a spot of blood on the yolk. When I returned to the table, my guest had changed the subject, now orating on the effort to unionize the adjuncts at his university—"the wrong union at the wrong time"—and the others continued to pretend to be paying attention, and I did my best to appear as though nothing unusual had just taken place.

4

No Big Deal

"**P**robably a UTI," says my GP. She phones in a prescription for Cipro. "Take these twice a day for ten days and you'll be okay." But I'm not okay. I watch the blood in the toilet bloom like one of those time-lapse photos of an exotic flower transformed from bud to blossom. Every morning I stand in front of the toilet praying for a stream the color of sunlight. For weeks it would be. Then the blood returns, like the first plague God visits upon the Egyptians in Exodus.

"I'm freaking out," Stacey tells her sister Amy on the phone when she thinks I'm not listening. She's in the bedroom, door shut, and I'm in the living room watching *The Wild Bunch* for the eleventh time, but the wall is thin and I've lowered the volume.

"The doctor says it's a remote possibility," Stacey says after a listening pause. "I've been googling—I know, I know, that way madness lies, but still.

"You mean, besides the blood in the urine?

"Lower back pain on one side (check, since the summer) and upper thigh and pelvic pain (check, he's had pain in his groin which he thinks was a muscle pull from too vigorous swimming).

"I'm a nervous wreck."

"Don't panic," Dr. Isamu says when the antibiotics fail to solve the problem, and sends me to Dr. Langsam, an expensive out-of-network urologist.

"The symptoms sometimes go away of their own accord, but that can be temporary," Dr. Langsam says. He avoids making eye contact. "The sample you left contained trace elements of blood."

"What does that mean? An infection?"

"Perhaps. The tests can be inconclusive. We sometimes get a false negative."

I'm wondering whom he reminds me of—I mean in looks. The young Bruno Ganz, maybe?

"You need a cystoscopy," he says, looking over his shoulder as he washes his hands. "I won't jolly you along—most men wouldn't volunteer to have one. That said, it's over quickly. Here I'll show you the apparatus."

This guy radiates confidence. "Men come from hundreds of miles away for my cystoscopies."

Maybe, but I almost pass out—from fear more than from pain—while the catheter is in me.

"You have a polyp—no big deal—but you'll need to have it scooped out," he says. He hands me the name and phone number of another urologist, a younger man, Dr. Caine. "Best surgeon in the city," he says, "for what you have."

"Which is?"

Cancer: so far no one has used the dread word, but I bring it up in Dr. Langsam's office. "It's unlikely," he says. "It's remote. But even if you have it, bladder cancer is one hundred percent curable if you catch it early." The double *if* undid the rest. I knew it then. *It was likely. It was not remote.*

A week later, I visit Dr. Caine for another cystoscopy.

More than what he said, I remembered the enthusiasm in the brilliant young doctor's voice when, after examining me, he announced, with the air of a mathematician who has solved a problem long thought insoluble, "You have bladder cancer."

5

Cancer Alley

Like every cancer patient on getting the bad news, I wondered what I had done to deserve this punishment. How does one even *get* bladder cancer?

"We don't really know," Dr. Caine said. "Have you ever taken the New Jersey Turnpike from the Holland Tunnel?"

I nodded.

"Then you've inhaled the fumes from all of those processing plants. You know what we call that stretch of highway?"

I make a stale joke about New Jersey's official moniker as the "Garden State."

"Cancer Alley," he says. "When the wind changes direction, you can be fifty miles away and you still inhale the toxins."

This is news to me.

"Do you live below Fourteenth Street?"

"Yes."

"Were you there on 9/11 and after?"

"Yes."

"Well . . ." His voice trailed off.

6

The Crisis

Wake up at four AM. Can't pee. I hold off telling Stacey for as long as I can but finally I waken her. She calls Dr. Caine, can't reach him. She calls Dr. Langsam and explains the situation to the answering service. We wait for a return call.

"Go to the ER," the sleepy voice says. "I can't do anything for you."

Stacey and I throw on yesterday's clothes and rush out. It's snowing. No, it's not just snowing, it's a full-fledged nor'easter, wind gusts and heavy wet snow. Two inches have already settled. We hail a cab, and just like Cary Grant and his secretary in *North by Northwest*, we push away the businessman with his hand on the handle. "Sorry," I say. "This is an emergency."

The ER at Beth Israel is relatively quiet though it won't be for long. Stacey has phoned my GP, who clears the way for me to be treated quickly upon our arrival. We are lucky because soon all available hands must attend to the victims of a bus and food truck collision on Fourteenth Street.

Dr. Pomerantz, the ER attending physician, is generous with an opioid. "This is payback for being a man," she says, handing me the pill and a prescription for more. She isn't smiling. "Now you can imagine what we women go through—menstruation, pregnancy, childbirth. Think of it."

A tabloid reporter turns up to interview the Hispanic man on one side of my privacy curtain. He has survived the deadly collision only because he had taken a seat in the very back of the bus. The driver was not so lucky. "I just thank God. I just thank God," the survivor keeps saying as a nurse picks out shards of glass from his leg. Several of his immediate family members crowd around.

On the other side of the curtain lies a barely coherent wino trying to answer a nurse's set questions.

"Did you drink today?"

"I did."

"How much?"

"Not sure."

"A bottle?"

"Yeah, a bottle."

7

The Aftermath

Robert Pinsky on the phone. "After six days, how did the catheter feel?"

"You really want to know?"

"Yes."

"Like a bayonet in my dick," I said.

What's more, the ER resident who jammed it in was new to this rotation. "You're my first catheter," he says, eager to try what had been until then an abstraction. He is like an inexperienced nurse who can't find a vein, jabbing over and over again until he forgets that a live person is on the receiving end. Soon he must call a colleague to assist. They work on me as if I'm a test dummy until finally the thing gets where it's supposed to go.

"No matter what the long-haired Buddhist full-of-shit poets write about flowers and rocks and clouds, you don't really understand life until you've had a Foley catheter stuck in you for six days," my friend Herb Engelhardt, an Okinawa veteran who has just turned ninety, says.

8

The Procedure

"Now that we know you have cancer, we have to determine how serious it is. In most cases—by most I mean seventy-five percent—we remove the growth and that's the end of it."

"What about the other twenty-five percent?"

"We have ways of treating it. But first things first."

The procedure is scheduled for eight AM the following Wednesday, which means I have to report to the hospital by five. The admissions waiting room is crowded though there's a general hush. A TV with the sound off is tuned to local news; a forecast of more snow appears in the crawl. Stacey tries to hold my hand, but I would rather distract myself by reading the sports pages and writing in my notebook.

While I am under general anesthesia, the surgeon will use a special instrument to look at my bladder and scrape out anything suspicious for the biopsy.

"It's a routine procedure," he says. Technically it's a TURBT—transurethral resection of bladder tumors.

Never believe a doctor when he or she says something is "routine."

9

The Protocol

The man, an overgrown boy, a naïf, a son, has a disease. There is a name for this disease. It is not a romantic name. He is too old to be a young romantic poet with the good sense to die in Rome on a winter day or at sea in a gale that he has commanded as a conductor flicks his baton and the woodwinds come to life. There was divinity in music that you could see like the notes floating above the piano in a Fauve painting.

Jessica, the nurse in charge of scheduling, is very nice and very matter-of-fact when issuing instructions on the day before the procedure. She wears standard-issue nurse's garb: pastel-blue baggy pants and a flowered smock-like shirt. Gone are the nun-like white dresses and caps of the nurses of my youth, the uniform that fueled a subgenre of romance novels.

"Here's the protocol. No food or anything after midnight. You may shower and brush your teeth."

Stacey is taking notes so I can tune out. The screen saver on the computer fades from a picture of a litter of golden retriever puppies to a field of wildflowers, then to an empty beach somewhere in the Mediterranean. Along the bottom a line of script announces that all of the pictures were taken by hospital staff.

"Wear something loose and comfortable. Leave jewelry at home. Yes, that includes wedding band. Noon, maybe sooner, it's a quick procedure. About forty-five minutes plus an hour to wake up and get stable. Release two PM. Could be earlier. Depends. You're very welcome, sir. Have a good one."

"You may take Valium with a sip of water," she says on her way out, but in my notebook I write, "You may take realism with a sip of water."

10

The Good Kind

When I arrive for the TURBT, I march into the operating room with the confidence of a world conqueror, joking with the nurses. The anesthesiologist, a young woman who appears to be the age of one of my graduate students, reviews some basic information. "This is just a blip," she says. "You'll be fine."

By blip she means it's not an automatic three-months-and-you're-out death sentence on the order of pancreatic cancer.

"If you're going to have cancer," she says, "this is the good kind."

When I wake in the recovery room, it is as if my unconscious wounded body has been brought in from the battlefield on a makeshift cot.

Stacey to Denise Duhamel: "We got the pathology report on Monday and unfortunately we didn't get the unqualified good news we were hoping for. David's cancer is 'aggressive/T1' which means it has invaded the bladder surface (though not the muscle, we hope). The dr. is going to repeat the surgery on April 18 to make sure he got it all and that it's 'graded' properly. From there we'll know what kind of treatment is best. Meanwhile David is having a CAT scan next Friday.

"Keep praying."

Three days after the scan you can expect to hear the results.

"It was basically okay," the doctor reports via e-mail. "There is a little abnormality in one bone, so maybe we should do a bone scan, but it could be an overread. Also, a very small solitary nodule in the lungs. so we should do a chest CT scan as well. But again I think an overread." If "overread" is shorthand for seeing something that isn't there, it helps drive home the point that medicine remains largely a matter of guesswork. After a while you figure out the lingo and decode the false optimism meant to boost patient morale. For example they say, "Oh, you can go back to work in two days," which is true only if the days are as long as in the first chapter of Genesis.

11

The Diarist

I will keep a diary and write in it every day. Everyone says I should but that's not the reason. The reason is—I am either a magician or an old dog, and this is not a new trick. I speak with bravado, though the real purpose of this project is to distract me from the facts of disease and death, and if there are truths along the way, so much the better.

And what, after all, is a diary? Why write twenty lines a day, let alone a prose poem? Are poems like vitamins or medications that you need to take daily? I'm not sure how to answer except to say that I have been writing in a pocket notebook every day for forty years. It's the single best thing a writer can do.

Columbia, 1969: According to Professor Edward Tayler, who called me "rhymester Lehman" in our seminar on seventeenth-century poetry, "there are two kinds of people in the world: those who divide everything in two, and those who don't." And you, my dear boy, are a Gemini, sign of the twins, Castor and Pollux, the Dioscuri, noted for their loyalty to each other and their elevator-like lives—one day in heaven, the next day in the other place. Pollux pleaded with Zeus to let him share his immortality—at the cost of halving it—with Castor killed in combat. Great warriors, stars vaulted into the midnight sky, whose fame is, however, surpassed by that of their twin half sisters, Clytemnestra and Helen of Troy. The former is the badass mother of militant feminism, who slew her husband, Agamemnon, the commander in chief, in the bathtub, while the latter launched a thousand ships, sparked the Trojan War, survived *The Iliad* and *The Odyssey*, went to Troy with Paris, and came back to be the Queen of Sparta and drink from her nightly flask of forgetfulness with her red-haired husband.

12

None But the Strong

D r. Kidder wore his version of a kindly smile. "You're in good physical condition, not overweight, your heart is normal, your blood pressure is in the safe zone. So we can proceed." He paused. "You see," he said, "we are going to mount an unprecedented assault on your person. None but the strong can take it." "And I'm strong?" "You are. Except for the cancer, you're in excellent health."

Student of rhetoric that I am, I thought of Marion Barry, the former mayor of Washington, who, when asked about criminal activity in the nation's capital, replied, "Outside of the killing, DC has one of the lowest crime rates in the country."

Meanwhile Dr. Kidder was joined by Dr. Schultig, his apprentice, and a guest oncologist from Johns Hopkins, Dr. Priyanka. To witness Drs. Schultig and Priyanka compete to win the approval of the older man was like watching two rivals for tenure serve as cointerviewers of the Nobel laureate from Peru, or like Gormley and Garrett vying for Commissioner Reagan's approval in *Blue Bloods*, an easy TV show to get addicted to when you're flat on your back. The young doctors were taller than Dr. Kidder and leaner and had more hair and I wondered what in private each would say about the other.

Stacey puts her research skills to the test and ascertains that bladder cancer is the sixth most common cancer among men. The biggest risk factor is smoking. It doesn't matter when you quit.

But, oh, did I love the smell of Gauloises and Gitanes at La Coupole or Le Dôme.

13

Tropic of Cancer

The tropic of cancer is a crowded waiting room, the doctor's running late, there's been an emergency, and people are wheezing or coughing or putting up a good front or looking bewildered, and you read a tabloid or a magazine, do a crossword puzzle, or bury your nose in *Tropic of Cancer*, Henry Miller's non-novel novel, which remains great though it has gone out of fashion, as politically incorrect now as it was in the 1950s but for radically different reasons. "Who wants a *delicate* whore! Claude would even ask you to turn your face when she squatted over the *bidet*. All wrong! A man, when he's burning up with passion, wants to see *everything*." In contrast, "Germaine had the right idea: she was ignorant and lusty, she put her heart and soul into her work. She was a whore all the way through—and that was her virtue!"

Suppressed for its sexual content in the 1960s, objectionable today on feminist or puritanical grounds, the stuff always was an example of brilliant writing. Note the grammatically liberating use of exclamation points in the few sentences I just quoted. Miller's rhetorical skill is at the service of passion on the one side and, on the other, the exploration of a whole realm of adult existence once thought to be alien to literature.

I'm grateful to Henry Miller for redeeming one lengthy session in the waiting room. Solzhenitsyn's *Cancer Ward* gets me through others.

Most weeks I don't bring a book. I don't carry a smartphone, a Kindle, an iPad, or any of these accessories, but I do have my notebook, and when I write in my notebook in the waiting room, it's as if I have closed my eyes in bed and can see myself from afar standing wearing a trench coat looking young at the baggage section of a Paris airport, de Gaulle or Orly, or maybe Stansted or Luton or Gatwick in England, way back when.

14

Hospitals and Airports

W hy do they go together in my mind, hospitals and airports? Because of the year I spent too much time in both—the year my father died in stages and I flew home twice from London, once from Paris. I have just turned twenty-three, am reading Hemingway and going to Pamplona with the gang, drinking wine from a pouch at the bullfight arena, getting hassled by the police for sleeping in a public park, there being no hotels or guesthouses with vacancies. Lew fakes an acid trip, convincingly. Then to Madrid and the Prado, the Valley of the Fallen, the cult of death, mussels with lemons, hot sauce and cerveza, paella and gazpacho, horchata and getting thrown out of the hotel for immoral conduct after Heidi and her lover quarrel and Mark shares her room chastely the next night. When the proprietor throws our bags down the stairs and calls the cops, suspecting us of whoring, Heidi hightails it to Barcelona; Lew and Mark, out of money, return to Paris, while Jamie and I take the train to Valencia and from there to Cerbère on the French border and then to Aix-en-Provence. We see *My Fair Lady* dubbed into French and have drinks with Slide Hampton and his trombone at the café with the blind saxophonist Michel Rocque, who, speaking English, sounds like a character in an Ionesco play: "We are very well here. We are very well here. So much the better!" Jamie captures the heart of Monica, a clever and lithesome California blonde, who locks him in her room after they spend the night together. Jamie is unfazed: *Vive la différence!* And Mont Sainte-Victoire sits grandly in the green background just as Cézanne rendered it. Gitane sans filter, carafe of red wine, and an impromptu pinball contest with a French Legionnaire who reeks of belligerence and is looking for a young man to subjugate.

For one who feels as out of step with his time as I do, the desire to go back, back in time, back home, is constant.

But there's no going back. There's no going backward in pleasure, as Kenneth Koch used to say in his lectures. There may be a few things you can recover but youth isn't one of them. *Youth.* There was a time when I associated the word with a phrase from Joseph Conrad: the romance of illusions. Now George Bernard Shaw's observation that youth is wasted on the young has become a self-evident axiom. I like the modern English adage: *If the old could, if the young knew.*

15

Back to the Waiting Room

Half the people won't shut up. The stocky man on his cell phone is so goddamn loud that another patient tries to quiet him and they almost come to blows. A woman is wailing. Two other women are talking up a tempest in a language I can't identify. Then a tall broad-shouldered guy, maybe an off-duty cop, gets on his feet and tells everyone to shut up. He says it with such authority that the rest of us stop what we're doing and look at him.

"Do you know what today is?" he says. No one answers. He raises his voice. "Today is the day they killed JFK."

In fact today is the third of March, but my mind flashes back to November 22, 1963, when the sixties, giddy with excitement, heroic and optimistic, the sixties of astronauts and glamorous center fielders, of Audrey Hepburn and "Moon River," James Bond, the Rat Pack, and the beehive hairdo, screeched to a halt. Before LBJ intervened in the Dominican Republic and intensified the war in Vietnam, committing more and more American troops, with the secretary of defense using a pointer and a blackboard to demonstrate why we would win the war in six months, the decade had felt like an extension of the fifties, not just the easy-to-caricature fifties of *Lassie* and singing cowboys on TV but the black-and-white fifties of Franz Kline's paintings or the Modern Jazz Quartet.

But Johnson succeeded Kennedy, Nixon took Johnson's place, the China opening on the plus side got canceled out by Watergate and OPEC on the negative, and there ensued the disastrous sequence of events that has led us to the wilderness. Condensed this way, history, our history, is a grief-stricken elegy, a nightmare recollected in an emergency. You might also consider it a mystery novel, the greatest unsolved murder of the century: the death of Kennedy, and the many conspiracy theories circling around it, which are continuous with the paranoia and, just below the surface, the panic that everyone in this room feels.

At an estate sale in Ithaca, I picked up a handsome 1963 wall calendar published by the Travelers Company in Hartford, Connecticut. In the room adjacent to our kitchen I hung it with November showing. There's a lithograph on the November page. It's called "Wild Duck Shooting" and it shows two men, two dogs, a rifle, and a scattering of fourteen wild ducks. No visitor to my house notices the calendar, though the room is one in which we spend much time and the calendar is prominently displayed. Everyone assumes it is current.

16

"Hurry up, please, it's time"

Have you read Aldous Huxley's novel *Time Must Have a Stop*? It is said he thought it the most successful of his attempts to fuse ideas with plot. A young man goes to Italy and gets educated by two mentors, one spiritual (a bookseller), the other a hedonist. There's a funny bit in which a deceased atheist returns in a séance and complains that his medium garbles his messages from beyond. But as a refutation of time it is not very convincing. Only in sports is it possible to stop the clock.

To write is to evade. I shall do my best to escape into memory and dream. And yet I also know that every time I put on a fedora and suspenders, suit and tie—every time I shave, as I stubbornly do, with a shaving brush and mug—what else am I doing but trying futilely to stop time?

17

Why 1963?

My aunt Esther, the emerita professor of philosophy, laughed with her old zest. "Don't give me that 'America lost its innocence' spiel," she said. "It's false in the precise way a cliché can be false. Alternative histories centering on November 22, 1963, are second only to conspiracy theories as invitations to the imagination. But the argument that November 22, 1963, marks the day when everything changed is a little too familiar, a little too easy, don't you think? Think of other dates when history changed just like that, a snap of the fingers." She refilled my cup and offered me another slice of the German poppy seed roll called Mohnstrudel, which I can never resist. We're sitting in her cluttered and somewhat shabby living room. She rearranged a pile of books and magazines on the coffee table to make room for the tea and cake.

I've been visiting Esther once a week for years. I did so at first out of a sense of obligation; she is my father's youngest sister, a widow, an intellectual starved for intelligent company, and before he died my father asked me to be good to her. Soon I looked forward to these visits as opportunities to try out my nascent ideas about history and politics, knowing that she would argue with me, not as an adult argues with a child, but as if I were an intellectual equal. As a boy, I thought of her as an elderly woman, though looking back I realize that she was probably younger by a couple of decades than I am now. She worked hard to rid herself of her German accent but it's obvious to me, especially when she relaxes and quotes Schopenhauer or Nietzsche. Had she been allowed to get a university education in Germany, she would have held an endowed chair at Harvard. But she was lucky to escape the Nazis and work at menial jobs while pursuing her degree at night at the New School. Now she must satisfy her formidable intellect by lecturing to young people at the community college who had heard it was a gut course.

"The fall of the Bastille," she said. "The assassination of Archduke Ferdinand in 1914. The day the stock market crashed in 1929. Or the otherwise unremarkable day in December 1910 when Virginia Woolf and a select group of friends had tea and a good frank discussion, and on that day human nature changed decisively. Marvelous, no? But utterly arbitrary. You can do better than 'America lost her innocence.'"

"All right: 1963 because I turned fifteen that year. And if a boy does not feel the call when he is fifteen, he appeals to the seminary of the world rather than that of saints, monks, holy men, and sacred objects."

"You lost your faith?"

"I kept kosher and observed the Sabbath until my second year at Columbia, but I never lost my faith."

"So you're a protestant Jew."

"I suppose you could say that. I head to the woods and read the Bible."

"What about politics?"

"My politics are like those of the character in Harry Mulisch's novel *The Assault* of whom it is said: 'Politics meant as little to him as a paper airplane to the survivor of a plane crash.'"

"What did happen when you were fifteen?"

- President Kennedy was assassinated while we were reading *The Odyssey* or *Robinson Crusoe* with an uninspiring teacher who patiently explained to the class that we were not only sophomores but also sophomoric. The previous spring Mr. Curran, an old theater man, made us memorize the speech Antony gives in *Julius Caesar* while standing over the body of Caesar—the speech that begins "O, pardon me thou bleeding piece of earth" and contains the phrase "the dogs of war." Mr. Curran played recordings of John Gielgud, Orson Welles, and Marlon Brando reading the lines. He made so strong a case for Brando's version that when Joseph L. Mankiewicz's 1953 picture (with Brando as Antony, Gielgud as Cassius, James Mason as Brutus, Greer Garson as Calpurnia, Deborah Kerr as Portia, and Louis Calhern as Caesar) was shown at the Arts Theater on Eighth Street, I took the subway all the way down from Dyckman Street to see it. I still know the speech by heart and strongly advocate memorization for its pedagogic value but don't get me started.
- During the winter holidays that year, my father and mother took me and my younger sister to Washington, DC. We stayed at the Ambassador, a hotel I picked from the travel section of the *Sunday Times*. As our blue 1962 Dodge Dart approached the entrance, I got out and asked a uniformed doorman if parking was free for guests. "Only the air is free in Washington, DC," he said. The hotel had a swimming pool. A girl from France was staying at the hotel with her family and I tried speaking French to her in the swimming pool. My father took us to see *Charade*. And in Italian restaurants he confidently ordered in Italian, which he learned when he lived in Milan in 1936 and '37. It was Italian with a German accent. Still, the waiters were impressed and we grinned with pride at my cosmopolitan papa. We ate manicotti and eggplant parmigiana and my parents shared a carafe of Chianti. This was unusual. Except for the Sabbath wine and obligatory four glasses at Passover, my parents rarely drank. One glass

in and mother's cheeks were bright pink and her laughter at my antics was heartier than usual. There are few greater pleasures to a boy than that of making his mother laugh. At the National Gallery we looked at the French impressionists. My father had a soft spot for "underrated ones, like Pissarro and Sisley," but favored Degas's dancers and bathers and Monet's haystacks, poplars, and cathedrals.

- In 1963 my next-door neighbor Joel and I developed the knock-knock system we used for the following four or five years. Two knocks on the wall separating our apartments meant we would meet on the fire escape. From our third-floor perch we enjoyed our view of the streets and especially the girls walking on them. Helen was the girl I liked the most. We called her "A." Joel was high on Ronnie, who was "B." The irony is that I thought it was Helen I fancied but it was really her younger sister Paulette. They lived on Seaman Avenue near its intersection with Cumming Street in Inwood.

- In 1963 Vietnam was the name on the canceled postage stamp Ivan Bass gave me in exchange for one of my Belgian beauties; cherry lime rickeys tasted good at Nat and Phil's, and miniature golf still seemed like a lot of fun.

- In 1963 for the first time I heard Frank Sinatra sing "I've Got You Under My Skin."

- On Good Friday 1963, Martin Luther King was jailed for protesting segregation in Birmingham, Alabama.

- In Game One of the 1963 World Series, Sandy Koufax outpitched Whitey Ford, and the Dodgers beat the Yankees in unheard-of fashion, four straight games. Johnny Podres, Ron Perranoski, and Don Drysdale were the only other pitchers the Dodgers needed in the sweep, with Koufax on the mound again for the finale. As a Dodger fan, proud of the team for breaking the color barrier in 1947 with Jackie Robinson, I was overjoyed.

18

Good Friday

The next procedure is scheduled for April 18, Good Friday and day four of Passover.

Each time I go to the hospital for a treatment, a shot, a test, a scan, or just an ordinary consultation, I can't help thinking of the last paragraph of George Orwell's essay "How the Poor Die" where he says that "the dread of hospitals probably still survives among the very poor and in all of us it has only recently disappeared. It is a dark patch not far beneath the surface of our minds." The wards remind Orwell of the "reeking, pain-filled" hospitals of the nineteenth century, and a "sickly smell" transports him back to a childhood illness in all its details. Now, to be sure, the hospitals in New York are clean, antiseptic, and artificially chilled. No "sickly smell" of imminent death and corruption. Yet it's there, that dread, that dark patch, whenever I enter one of the many buildings in the cancer complex. I have checked my professional and personal identity at the door and am now just an ordinary ailing human specimen, male.

Here comes Geiger, the ward psychologist slash social worker. He wants me to talk about my dreams, my fears, my psyche, whatever, but I don't want to talk, so he tells doctor jokes. "The bad news is you're going to die. The good news is I'm fucking my nurse." "You want a second opinion? You're ugly, too." Also knock-knock jokes. "Sam and Janet Who?" "Sam and Janet Evening." "How many flies does it take to screw in a lightbulb? Two, but I don't know how they got in there." I contribute one from the mimeographed scandal-sheet-cum-Dadaist-single-page-publication that the fellows at *Columbia Review* put out sporadically in 1968 and '69. On a Friday afternoon the rabbi bought a live chicken for the Shabbat dinner, but there was still time so he went to the movies, hiding the bird in his trousers. The girl sitting next to him elbowed her girlfriend. "Ah, you've seen one, you've seen them all," the friend said. "But this one's eating my popcorn!" The headline: "Rabbi's Pecker Freaks Out Chicks."

Freud would have had no problem elucidating the deep meaning of each of these except perhaps the one about "Some Enchanted Evening." I bring up Freud and his joke book and Geiger says he has never read Freud but knows that Freud and Willie Mays share a birthday, May 6.

19

Lasciate ogni speranza, voi ch'entrate!

There are those who make cancer the sun around which the rest of the planets revolve. They read voraciously, they join support groups, they research the available options, they buy the right vitamins and herbs, they know what ingredients to look for on the label of a soft-drink bottle, they go to an acupuncturist, they avail themselves of the Cancer Resource Center, they go to the Internet. They want to know everything—the treatments, the chance of a cure, the medications and their side effects, what a TURBT feels like, how a Foley catheter differs from the kind they use in immunotherapy, what you can expect to have happen in chemo. Not me. I don't want to talk about it, think about it, do anything about it except show up on time for every last appointment and try not to complain. Luckily Stacey is willing to do the research for the both of us, and the worrying.

I know I should read the books about cancer that well-meaning people have bought for me—especially the highly touted ones with "journey" in the title. But first I must practice breathing into this funny device that has a name that sounds like percolator. Is it speculator? No, it's spirometer, "an instrument for measuring air inhaled into and exhaled out of the lungs, providing a simple way of determining lung volume and capacity." Okay, I'll practice breathing. But I refuse to utter or write the words "my cancer journey" as if I were on a soft-focus adventure to the land of wellness.

What I am entering is a gate and on the top of the gate is written, in three languages, *"Lasciate ogni speranza, voi ch'entrate! Vous qui entrez ici, abandonnez toute espérance.* Abandon all hope, ye who enter here." I'd rather go to hell with Dante as my guide or do anything else with my so-called free time than see another doctor or read another page about this disease that no one wants, which it is impossible to glamorize (unlike the consumption that brought down Keats or even the venereal disease that caused some nineteenth-century prophets to lose their minds), and which (despite Susan Sontag's efforts) remains a term for evil—like Fascist. The other day I heard a portly politician shout hoarsely against the "cancer of income inequality." I remember when Ronald Reagan said, "I didn't have cancer. I had a part of me that had cancer and I had that part removed."

In the weeks before the first symptoms showed up, I read Tolstoy's *Death of Ivan Ilych*, Lionel Trilling's *Middle of the Journey*, and Dante's *Inferno*—a tale of impending death, a near miss that causes the protagonist to rethink everything, and a vision of what may await us after the Reaper comes to claim his due. What the unconscious knows ahead of time.

20

The Weekend Before

He was in Miami, South Beach, the weekend before the first symptoms manifested themselves. This is what he wrote in his journal.

Go to the swimming pool, small, not even a quarter Olympic size. There are three grown palms and a sapling for company. There's blessed silence for the count of ten and then you hear "I Heard It Through the Grapevine." Fine song but you'll get no reading done here. You're about to start chapter four and you identify yourself strongly with the hero, who is thirty-three years old and recovering from a near brush with death on account of a freak illness. What did the experience teach him? He grew to distrust any secular ideologue with the possible exception of Freud. Women interested him—their conversation, their long hair, their vanity: the hoops or little garnet earrings, the pearl necklace, the heels, the sunglasses of the rich and hungover. Our hero had spent two months in the care of Nurse Gillian, a tough-love Englishwoman with a matter-of-fact demeanor who tolerated his flirtation with the idea of death for the time it took for a bouquet of roses to bloom, wither, and die. Then she put her foot down. It was time to leave the hospital. *Il faut tenter de vivre.* He is unmarried, his fiancée having succumbed to pneumonia the previous winter. Their love affair had been a lucky chance snatched by fate. You are in his mind as he resigns himself to the loss, to being a loner, but you are also at the pool where a ballad for the sad world in the form of a folk song with harmonica is driving you nuts. There's a mirror across the pool where the inconspicuous body attired in an aqua blue tennis shirt is visible. The Supremes take over: "You Can't Hurry Love."

He undertook a self-appraisal. He had done well in his chosen field before his close call with death from which with manly stoicism he was recovering, having lost his youth in the interim. What could he do? He couldn't jump up and down and try to strangle the Fates for taking her away. He had once wanted to be great, to be famous, and that time now was gone. But something could still be done. He had almost died with "Ode to a Nightingale" on his lips—something only a professor of English writing a novel would do.

Go to the beach, try to ignore the bikinis, God bless them. Why some of us are so enamored of strategically concealed female flesh is like the green waves turning white as they crash on the shore. People pass. At least they have the good manners to speak in a foreign language. I would like to paint the waves, the waves and also the bathers, lying on chaises under orange and light-green and navy-blue umbrellas—dotting the beach in democratic delight. And the little kids climbing the crest of a wave, or diving into it, or riding with it to the shore as I did in Far Rockaway when I was eleven.

All afternoon: the image of "The Swimmer"—or is it called "The Bather"—by Cézanne at the Museum of Modern Art. That is who I am, staring at the sea head down arms akimbo or just shrugging my shoulders listening to the waves at night when no one else is around.

21

"Bladder cancer: Isn't that what Sinatra died of?"

Like the March TURBT, the same procedure in May was considered a success. It looked like they got all the bad stuff out of his insides. In the summer he endured eight weeks of BCGs, an immunotherapy regimen in which a bacillus is injected directly into the bladder.* (Don't ask how.) The patient was still cancer-free in September. This was confirmed by a cystoscopy from the one doctor who insisted on conversing while the procedure was going on.

"You're good for now," he said, but you could tell a "but" was coming.

"No buts. There's always a chance with high-grade cancer that it will return, but you knew that."

"And if it does come back?"

"As long as it doesn't penetrate the bladder wall, you're okay."

Okay, he was okay, and that summer he hurried to complete on deadline his book on Frank Sinatra. It was thrilling to write every day. He was on fire. Even when he wrote that Sinatra died of bladder cancer, very painfully, he didn't take it to heart. But from time to time he felt a pain in his midsection, sometimes when walking,

---

* Bacillus Calmette-Guérin (bovine tuberculosis bacillus).

sometimes after swimming, and one day in October he fell down half a flight of steps. At night he felt fatigued, weak.

The cystoscopy revealed the bad news. The tumor had returned. And there was no time to lose. A procedure, his third TURBT in nine months, preceded by a CT scan, took place four days later. The verdict: the cancer had metastasized. They didn't inform him right away; they let his wife bring him the message when he was drugged and drowsy and just regaining consciousness after twenty-four hours of sheer oblivion.

22

In a Technical Sense

After the operation, Stacey sat in a private room waiting to be briefed by the doctor. The room resembled a small living room, with two love seats flanking a low coffee table. When the doctor entered he took the seat farthest away from her, not on one of the love seats but in the chair nearest the door. The common touch he didn't have.

"In a technical sense," the doctor said, "your husband died. But only for six seconds. In a technical sense," he repeated.

When I came to, I heard I had had a heart "block."

"You're a lucky man," the doctor said.

"I am?" I said.

"You're lucky this happened here." He spread out his arms as if to say: look at all we can do to keep you alive.

But the significance of his statement was lost on me as I returned to my dream and checked out of hearing range.

I died a second time, for just four seconds this time, and after they brought me back, they put me under with morphine and fed my sleeping body through my veins.

When I woke, my wife told me that the cancer had spread and that my aunt Esther had passed. I said: "Anything else?"

23

Five O'Clock Rush

The doctor left at five o'clock. My heart stopped beating at 5:01. There was no one in the room when I died and no one to notice the miracle of my return to consciousness. Perhaps you have heard of such cases. Someone has died, for all intents and purposes, then comes back to life. It happened to the composer Jerome Kern, for example, back in 1937.

But there was something unusual in my case. When I died it was one minute past five. When I woke the clock said 10:40, darkness had fallen outside, the radio was playing an old Sinatra song, "Young at Heart."

And here is the best part. When the song ended, the voice on the radio was the voice of the nurse, Alice, who differed from every other nurse in this purgatorial hospital by speaking to you not as if you were a child, not in the first-person-plural ("How are we feeling today?"), but in the hippest jive imaginable in 1948, June 1948, in the streets and alleys of downtown New York.

For that was the month and year in which I came to life, and this was the place. And here is the strange part. When I looked out the window I saw Alice, only now her name was Angel, in her customary raincoat in the customary drizzle walking into the street. Her back was turned to me. The studio was undecided between

Joan Fontaine and Ida Lupino for the part. But when I looked in the mirror I knew she was there with me in the room—I saw her standing there behind me grinning, naked, and reveling in the effect of her wild brown curls on my overheated imagination. I had turned nineteen that summer.

So I turned around a second time and saw the bed was made with her inside, naked except for her wild brown curls, and there was a night-light and a selection of books on the night table. Proust as rendered by Scott Moncrieff, *Anna Karenina* as translated by David Magarshack, Thomas Mann's *Joseph and His Brothers*, all four volumes in an old translation. And a spy novel: "The German minister smoked a Turkish cigarette in a jade holder. 'Nothing ever happens in Brussels,' he shrugged."

Not a bad way to go. And she was singing to me, my pear-shaped queen of diamonds, my Gibson with chips of ice like little islets on the surface of the liquid, and this was no hospital at all but a hotel, a grand hotel, and there was nothing stopping me from getting my old tuxedo pressed, sewing a button on my vest, because I had to look my best as I headed out for a night on the town. That's what I was doing. The clock said 4:20. I couldn't account for the intervening time. But I knew she'd be there when I got back.

24

A Heart Event

"This is not a zero-sum game," the surgeon said to the anesthesiologist. That's the last thing I remember before going under.

"You had a heart event," the nurse said. I nodded but in fact I had forgotten. The anesthesiologist came into the room and asked accusingly, "How come your heart stopped?"

"It hurts," I said, "like a son of a bitch."

"Where?"

"Below the belt."

"In the pelvic area," she corrected. Then she said, "That's why your heart stopped. The heart does not like pain."

"You were loopy," the nurse said when I woke up twenty-four hours later.

"What was the first thing I said that made sense?"

"You said, 'Won't anyone tell me where I am?'"

Coming back to life and consciousness, the mind knows it has been somewhere but is otherwise a blank, no dreams except life itself. "I have seen the future. It is the present but we are invisible. There is no honor in being old. Merely to have survived is no guarantor of virtue or wisdom or anything but luck."

Heroism is over. "These rare souls set opinion, success, and life at so cheap a rate that they will not soothe their enemies by petitions, or the show of sorrow, but wear their own habitual greatness." Emerson believed in heroes and trusted that God would make him happy.

But I chose the model of a Japanese poet who could make a tanka out of a pear, a knife, a tabletop, a tablecloth, and a tree shedding leaves in the window. I sat for a long time, every so often looking at my watch. I loved my watch not because I needed to know the time but because it had an intimate relationship to my wrist.

25

Good Show

In the hospital, where he had to spend the next four days, his head was too cloudy for the news to sink in. A few days after his release, the oncologist phoned.

"With one chemo regimen the best I can offer you is a fifty-fifty chance. With the other there's a very strong possibility of eliminating the cancer totally. Now which do you want?" He sipped from his Starbucks cup, thinking, "I expect you to answer in the next thirty seconds because I am about to go on holiday, which I have delayed, because as you see I have made you a top priority."

The patient gave the right answer.

"Good man! Of course the side effects are more severe. But it's only four or five months."

The patient thought about William Holden in *The Bridge on the River Kwai*, blackmailed by the stiff-upper-lip British officer to return to the Japanese prisoner of war camp from which he has risked life and limb to escape. "As long as I'm hooked I may as well volunteer," Holden says, and even jokes about the airborne assignment when he is told that he will have to forgo the customary practice run before making the jump. "With or without parachute?" he asks straight-faced. The British officers laugh, and the commander exclaims, "Good show, jolly good show."

26

Metaport

Regular access to his veins was necessary for the chemo infusions. If the needle goes into your arms, they will resemble a junkie's in no time. Much wiser to have the medics install a metaport in the chest: a device with a built-in catheter that needs to be flushed once a month but is much easier on the patient in the long run because the doctor or nurse is spared having to search for a vein and because the needle there is less painful.

For this next procedure, he reports fasting at nine for an eleven AM surgery. Per nurse Jessica's instructions, he has eaten nothing and drunk nothing for the previous twelve hours. Stacey has brought her knitting, he has the newspaper. Strategically placed signs ask visitors to refrain from eating or drinking out of consideration for the patients who are unable to do so while waiting to be called for surgery. The hours crawl by, one o'clock, two o'clock, three. They still haven't called him. He sleeps in the crowded noisy waiting room—he is in an airport now and keeps losing his luggage at baggage claims. He's the forlorn passenger beside the carousel with the suitcases and backpacks. One by one his fellow travelers have collected their belongings and departed for home. Some are greeted by their shrieking children and indulgent spouses who maintain calm despite the relief that their loved one has arrived safely. Others pull their luggage to the curb, where a limo awaits. A lone suitcase, held together with duct tape and rope, circulates hopefully, then tips over. Now he's the luggage that nobody wants. And he has a plane to catch, he has to go to work, but where is his briefcase, the leather one that his mother gave him? At four they wake him. Though still unwilling to admit to a scheduling snafu, they have found him an empty office with a computer so he can send off a few messages into the ether. He checks the market, then the ball scores. Stacey dozes on the recliner. At 5:30 he is on the operating table. The anesthetic wears off in the middle of the operation, and he has an amiable chat with the surgeon putting the finishing touch on his incision. Dr. Siegenthaler is one cheerful fellow. It turns out he did his undergraduate work at Yale then attended medical school at Columbia and even took Alan Ziegler's course in prose poems and other short literary forms. "Here, have a graham cracker and a can of orange juice," says an eager volunteer once the patient is wheeled into recovery. He hates graham crackers.

27

If You Were an English Poet

When I have the energy, when the chemo does not overwhelm me with fatigue, I write poems—or lines, not poems; sentences, observations, banter, similes, titles, notes to myself, all the stuff that goes into my pocket notebook.

Clive James, who has cancer, knows he is dying and writes about it. He, too, hates the medical and pharmaceutical terminology. Inevitably, he writes in "Procedure for Disposal," one of the poems in *Sentenced to Life*, he will "succumb / To these infirmities I'm slow to learn / The names of lest my brain be rendered numb / With boredom even as I toss and turn." I show the poem to Stacey and she says, "If you were an Australian poet living in Cambridge, this is what you'd write."

It is not just the illness but the constant reminder of your mortality that gets to you. It is no sure thing that you will recover from the cancer even if you survive the poison you take to kill it. The knowledge that you could die sooner than you expected—that's the shock you have to absorb.

The chance that you're on death row, with the date of execution up to the whim of a bureaucrat, makes you visit and revisit the past in order to make sense of it or to judge what you did or to weigh its significance or to speculate on how you will change your behavior if you do survive. I just reread that sentence and realize that the metaphors imply that to live is to commit a crime. Well, yes, to the extent that death is the ultimate truth and maybe the only one, we transgress every day we're alive. And a night in the hospital is like a day in prison. You lose track of the days. You know they will never let you go.

28

The Regimen

Words you never want to hear in the same sentence: high grade, aggressive, and rare.

My cancer was high grade, aggressive, and rare, with clear cell features in the lining. They warned me about the side effects of the chemo right from the start: nausea, dizziness, fatigue, neuropathy, and your immune system is compromised, so you never leave the house without gloves and you never take the subway. Avoid crowds and public places. No fast food, nothing raw, nothing greasy. No sushi, no pizza. No buffets. You'd be surprised how many chemo patients contract an infection, which could upset or prolong the treatment.

"And what if I get an infection, and how will I know?"

"You'll know."

"And then?"

"Then you head straight up to our 24/7 emergency room."

"Anything but that," I thought. There was incentive enough to play by their rules.

Three chemicals will get pumped into your "power port" for four months. Has Jasmine gone over the side effects with you? Very well, then. You know roughly what to expect. It may wreak havoc, but that's how we kill the cancer. Unfortunately we kill a lot of healthy cells, too. There is no way to distinguish between them. The oft-used simile for chemotherapy is the bombing of a whole city to knock out one building.

Can you be more specific?

Six cycles of three weeks each. Wednesday, Thursday, Friday, Saturday: dexamethasone (dex), five four mg. tablets on the night before and the morning of chemo; three four mg. tablets on days two, three, nine, and ten. Two straight Thursdays: cisplatin, carboplatin, paclitaxel. Every other Friday: Neulasta shot to ward off infections.

When you get a kidney infection, we will give you ceftriaxone intravenously, Zosyn (piperacillin/tazobactam) intravenously, and Cipro upon discharge. For painful urination: phenazopyridine. For your stomach: pantoprazole. For diarrhea: cholestyramine. For constipation: Colace. For C. diff: vancomycin and, when that doesn't work, Dificid.* For pain: Percocet, Vicodin, but you won't like these. For the endoscopy: propofol. For bronchitis: benzonatate. And don't forget the lidocaine. You will need to see two oncologists, five urologists, a neurologist, two cardiologists, an internist, a gastroenterologist, a dermatologist, two wound specialists, and a podiatrist before we're through with you.

Please arrive fasting. The procedure is scheduled for ten AM but will not start until five o'clock in the afternoon but that is because of a delay. "But that's the second time this has happened to me." We can explain. This is a hospital and emergencies happen. You have to let go of the belief that you are in control. You're not. Oh, you don't have to apologize for losing your temper. In your shoes I would do the same.

"Now stand tall for me, please," the nurse said.

---

* C. diff is shorthand for Clostridium difficile (C. difficile).

29

A Few Beacons in the Quicksand

"My father and mother didn't belong to any particular milieu," Nobel laureate Patrick Modiano writes in *Pedigree: A Memoir.* "So aimless were they, so unsettled, that I'm straining to find a few markers, a few beacons in this quicksand, as one might attempt to fill in with half-smudged letters a census form or administrative questionnaire."

Here are a few such markers for my uprooted parents, unsettled as they were, though far from aimless. You will have to make allowances for the lack of specific detail. Neither my father nor my mother would talk much about their lives before they landed on American shores, when he was twenty-seven and she twenty-three. It was as though they were reborn in the United States on the day they met in Manhattan, or the day they were married by Rabbi Breslauer three Sundays after Pearl Harbor, or the day their status as refugees formally ended and they became naturalized citizens with kids who were American by birth and could speak English better than they could.

I have the passports documenting the exact day my parents escaped from Germany and Austria, in 1936 and 1938, respectively. Josef Isaak Lehmann went, ostensibly on business, from Germany to France, where his cousin Martha lived with her husband in

Paris. A few months later he joined his sister and her husband in Milan. The summers at Lake Como were the happiest my father had ever known. There were young women aplenty and the tempo of life was so much more relaxed than in his native Fürth or nearby Nuremberg with its scary Heilig-Geist-Spital, which he knew all too well from his bout of rheumatic fever as a boy. In Italy, he felt as a high bourgeois character in a Thomas Mann novel does upon taking his holiday in the warm south. With his damaged heart, Joe did not find it easy to gain admittance to the United States, though he liked to point out that he shared his first name with Joe DiMaggio, the best ballplayer in America. This would prove that he could speak English and knew what's what. Cuba was less selective than the States in admitting displaced Europeans. Starting December 12, 1938, my father lived in Havana. About the year that followed I never heard him speak a word, though one day he startled me by speaking fluent Spanish on the phone with a customer in Caracas. In December 1939, on his second try, he entered the United States, which happened only because of the leniency and kindness of an immigration official in Florida. Maybe he was a Yankee fan.

Anna Lusthaus, Anny to her friends, lived on Friedmanngasse in Vienna. She was as lighthearted as her husband was serious. In Vienna she, high-spirited, carefree, with her brother Bert and their cousins Rita and Bina, played street games and parlor games, went dancing, acted in amateur theatricals, and listened happily to the tenor of the day, Josef Schmidt. Each of them followed a different itinerary from Vienna to New York. My mother was still in Vienna after the Anschluss in March 1938 when the Nazis annexed Austria, troops marched in, and welcoming swastikas hung from the windows of the enthusiastic Viennese. The Jews were forced to wash the sidewalks and paint yellow stars in their shop windows.

Longtime friends from school days suddenly shunned my mother in the street. Even after she lined up a sponsor in London, it took her months to obtain the necessary visas for leaving Austria. According to her passport, with the giant capital "*J*" signifying *Jude* in pink overshadowing the largest other words on the page, "*Reisepass*" and "*Deutsches Reich,*" Anny entered the United Kingdom on September 23, 1938. She worked as a parlor maid and part-time cook, first in Bournemouth and then in London. On November 23, 1939, Thanksgiving Day, she arrived in New York. She and my father met for the first time a year later at a social gathering for refugees where my father gallantly offered my mother his seat. Courting her, he took her to the movies and treated her to an ice cream soda afterward, spending a week's wages on the date, though he never let on. After seeing her home, he walked the whole way back to his furnished room, two and a half miles away.

Joseph Lehmann dropped the final *n* in his last name. In New York he held a few managerial positions and then, with the contacts he made, set up his own shop importing and exporting steel parts—beams, angles, reinforcing bars. My mother suggested he take the last three letters of his last name and the first two letters of his first name and thus was born the Manjo Steel & Trading Company. At 220 Broadway and later at 114 Liberty Street, he had an office separated by a glass partition from where his secretary sat and typed. The nicest of his secretaries was Margaret. Frieda did not like typing his son's high school term papers.

Joseph Lehman was elected president of Congregation Ohav Sholom, a position he took with great seriousness. He threw himself into the work. It gave him *nachas* but also *tsuris* and made me permanently wary of synagogue politics. The congregation consisted almost exclusively of Holocaust refugees and their American children. Like my father, Louis Kissinger came from Fürth, near

Nuremberg, in northern Bavaria. In the old country he taught history and geography. Here he was a retired bookkeeper who lived nearby in Washington Heights. He was older than my father, but they had Fürth and Judaism in common, and on some Saturdays after services, the two men would walk together in Fort Tryon Park, comparing the achievements of their sons. Henry had gone from Harvard to work at the White House and was still very devoted to his mother, Paula.

Soft-spoken but strict, my father observed every jot and tittle of the religious law—and gloried in the observance, be it the blessing you say upon seeing a rainbow or the ritual of searching on Passover eve for *chometz,* any trace of the foodstuffs forbidden to eat during the eight days of the holiday commemorating the exodus from bondage in Egypt. At our house we had four sets of plates: one set for dairy, one for meat, the third for Passover dairy, the fourth for Passover meat. To be an observant, intelligent, enthusiastic, and above all religious Jew—to be *frum*—was a full-time job. Between the Torah and the Talmud, the family and the office, the festivals and the fast days, where was the time for art? My father took courses in painting at the New School, but nothing came of that. There wasn't time enough in a life that a diseased heart would cut short.

My father knew he was going to die. A heart attack alerted him. But death frightened him, he associated doctors with death, he refused to have experimental surgery when he was younger, and his health began to fail around the time I left for England upon graduation from Columbia. In December he underwent open-heart surgery. A few months later he contracted jaundice, which we now call hepatitis C. In December he had a heart attack and I got on an emergency flight from Paris but was somewhere over the Atlantic when he died. So we never had certain conversations.

30

What's the Story?

Forgive the interruption, but what's the story? That's what my aunt Esther would say if she were still with us.

You need a story line in a novel or a movie. Surely I don't need to explain this to someone who reads books for a living! You have written, and I think I quote you exactly, that the absence of plot in a novel is as self-defeating as the absence of melody in music. And central to any story, as you very well know, is some sort of conflict and some surprising change of fortune or change in character. Quaker bride marries strong silent marshal but disapproves of violence until confronted with evil that won't go away unless met with resolute defiance. Hotshot hero comes home from the war but can't find work, and his wife is stepping out on him. Three army buddies vow to get together in ten years, and they do, but the facts of social and economic class have asserted themselves and the boys no longer like one another. The obstinate British colonel wins his battle of ego and will with the Japanese commander of the POW camp—only to turn around and help build the bridge that the enemy sorely needs. Does the adulterous candidate for governor renounce his ambition or destroy his marriage when his opponent threatens to reveal the love nest? That's what you need: a plot designed to get you to wonder what will happen next.

Your life as a movie. Will you play it straight—cancer and then treatment, an ordeal, the love of a loyal and capable spouse, some act of glory, and then what? Death? Recovery? Is it a medieval romance—a test, a quest, and a journey? A test of his will to live, the quest for a cure, a journey to a hospital across the country? Does the protagonist abandon the false values he once held dear? Does he denounce and renounce in the manner of Job who knows his terrible fate is unjust or Timon of Athens who generously lent money to everyone, forgave all debts, but found himself friendless when he lost his fortune and now he sits on a park bench and raises his fist and snarls at the passersby? Do the doctors give him six months, maybe nine, and does he return to the village where he grew up and imagine being the boy that he was then? Does he quit his job and move to the big city and get mixed up with high rollers and fast dames until his luck runs out and he is a wino on a Philadelphia sidewalk? Does he go to an old-fashioned red sauce Italian restaurant in the Village and get mistaken for a man he looks like, whose identity he assumes?

But I refuse to research the novel I am not writing. I don't know how the ordeal is going to turn out, and the road connecting memory and desire is not a linear path but a series of quick right and left turns dictated by the local authorities somewhat whimsically to regulate the flow of traffic. Glen, my literary agent and boon companion, thinks I should write an anatomy of cancer on the model of an *Anatomy of Melancholy.* But one lesson of any brush with death is that time is finite, and if you have gotten a reprieve and time is still on your side, you must do what you want and only that.

31

Time Is on My Side

Yes, it is, or was, or still is when I escape into that land of un-likeness. I wake in the morning and it is 1962, the year before the year the world changed utterly.

In 1962 the Mets came into existence and my father and I watched them drop a doubleheader to the Dodgers on Memorial Day at the Polo Grounds. Koufax pitched game one, Johnny Podres game two, for the erstwhile bums of Brooklyn, now playing for Los Angeles. It was a good day for the shortstops. Maury Wills of the Dodgers hit an inside-the-park home run. Elio Chacón of the Mets turned a triple play.

After each Mets game on the radio, a dramatic voice would say, "This is Howard Cosell, with big Ralph number thirteen Branca, speaking of sports." Branca was famous for throwing the pitch that the Giants' Bobby Thomson hit for the home run that ended the winner-take-all third game of the 1951 National League playoff between the New York Giants and the Brooklyn Dodgers—the moment that marked the all-time climax of baseball as the national pastime.

I graduated from the yeshiva in 1962. *The Carpetbaggers* was an eye-opener, full of girls walking in on boys with hard-ons and dreams of making money: oil fields, airplanes, and the design of

a bra capacious enough to hold the beauteous bombshell's boun-
tiful breasts. It was the American dream in a cup. In September
I entered Stuyvesant High School in the old building with its dis-
tinctive smells (jockstraps, sulfuric acid) at Fifteenth Street and
First Avenue.

In 1962 I no longer wore a cap in the street. I had sported a
Brooklyn Dodgers baseball cap in 1957 and LA caps from 1959
until 1961. I had felt safer, less self-conscious, wearing a baseball
cap rather than a yarmulke when I went to the yeshiva.

On the last night in June, Sandy Koufax pitched a no-hitter
in Dodger Stadium against the Mets. The next morning, a Sun-
day, my friend Saul phoned to congratulate me. Saul, with whom
I fought and played from the time we were seven years old, was a
big Yankee fan. His full name was Saul Solomon. The biblical Saul
was the king of Israel before David, and Solomon was David's son.
We played with the idea that my friend, a year younger than I, was
my rival on the one hand and my son and heir on the other.

Saul argued for Solomon, the fount of wisdom, whom God
chose to build the holy temple. I conceded that Solomon was wiser
and more pacific, but maintained that David was the greater hero
because he slew Goliath, he used a slingshot and geometric knowl-
edge to defeat a bigger opponent, and because the prophet Samuel
anointed him; because he enchanted King Saul with his harp play-
ing, because he mated with Bathsheba, because he committed in-
fidelities, because he stole another man's wife, and also because he
led Israel to military victory; because Saul had slain his thousands
but David his tens of thousands, and still today at every merry
function the kids in the synagogue's youth group sing, *"Dovid me-
lech Yisrael; chai, chai, vekayam"* ("David, king of Israel, lives and
endures"). And furthermore, because David had to escape from
Saul's jealous wrath, because David and Saul's son Jonathan loved

each other, because David's son Absalom rebelled against him, because David fasted and prayed when one of his sons was mortally ill, and when news of the lad's death reached him he ate a hearty meal because there was no point in fasting and praying after the fact. And finally because David was not only a man of action and a lover, he was also a poet, author of the psalms, and God protected him in the cave of his hiding as he protected Jacob on the night when the angels went up and down the ladder to heaven and Jacob slept within a circle of rocks, and because he prayed and had the faith that David put into words: *Yea, though I walk through the valley of the shadow of death, I will fear no evil: for thou art with me; thy rod and thy staff they comfort me.*

It was the summer of Ray Charles, "You Don't Know Me" and "I Can't Stop Loving You."* It was the autumn of Tony Bennett, "I Left My Heart in San Francisco," as the Giants beat the Dodgers for the pennant but lost to the Yankees in the Series—the 1951 scenario all over again. The Four Seasons broke out with "Sherry" and on the first day of music class the teacher said he was going to play the "Four Seasons" and the boys giggled when it turned out to be Vivaldi. There were three girls I liked but I didn't do anything about it except say their names in my prayers before going to sleep, praying that these pretty girls would find me as attractive as I found them. I put on *tefillin* every day and said my morning prayers. In those days I had a close relationship with the Lord.

In 1962, John Glenn orbited the earth three times. And on an October day, the subway station at First Avenue and Fourteenth Street, the station nearest Stuyvesant, was deserted except for me

---

* Some believe that the number-one song on the hit parade when you turn fourteen holds the key to your personality. Ray Charles and "I Can't Stop Loving You" were on top of the list in June 1962.

and a well-dressed woman in her forties. There were Soviet missiles in Cuba, and last night Kennedy vowed to intercept any Russian ship approaching the island.

"Do you think we're in for a nuclear war?"

"No," I said. "I think the Russians will back down. What do you think?"

"Let's hope you're right." In my diary I wrote a note warning my future self against nostalgia: "Remember misery of gym class, October 16, 1962."

32

Rush Job

Hospitals and airports. In dreams one stands for death, the other for life, the life of jeopardy. My girlfriend accompanied me to the airport. I had just flown in from a more or less leisurely assignment in France and now, after eight hours in her Brooklyn Heights apartment, I needed to cross the country, report, and write a rush story. Reba, that was her name, and I kissed at the gate. She was being as dramatic as possible, which is the way she was, her job at Credit Suisse notwithstanding.

"I bet you crash tonight," she whispered.

"That's a hell of a thing to say to a man about to board a plane," I answered.

What she had in mind was not a plane in flames but an exhausted man falling asleep as soon as his head hit the pillow. But somehow our relationship never recovered from this premonition of disaster. The story I was working on? About a hoax centered on Nazi memorabilia and pages from a diary said to be in Hitler's handwriting; it got exposed in Pasadena thanks to a bearded old man with a Viennese accent. In those days at airports I reminded myself that I worked in journalism, with datelines from Los Angeles, London, Paris, and New York, and I deserved that Tanqueray martini after packing it in at eight o'clock.

33

Final Call

Her name was Amy. She was one of the scores of baby boom girls named after Ray Bolger's rendition of "Once in Love with Amy" on Broadway. On a good day she looked like the young Shelley Winters playing opposite John Garfield in *He Ran All the Way*. At the airport we kissed good-bye. I must have looked exhausted.

"I'll bet you crash tonight," she said.

"That's a hell of a thing to say to a guy who's about to board a plane," I said, jauntily.

"You know what I meant," she said.

I did and tumbled headfirst into a dream in which I had to let her go, give her up, walk away, and console her when she burst into tears. I had underestimated the power of her tears, and how contagious they were—how, when I was alone, I too cried, not so much for her as for the feelings she inspired. "There will come a day when you wake up forgetting you were supposed to be sad," my mother consoled me. I was wearing corduroy trousers, a thick woolen sweater, warm socks, an Oxford University scarf. There was no central heating in England, so I translated a poem by Pierre Reverdy called "Central Heating." The woman in the blue silk dress and jade earrings spoke in an accent I had heard before. "Do you have a woman?" she asked. Afterwards we talked in whispers. The question was: Would you risk your life to save this person loved so briefly, and known in one way only? Birds filled the sky like afterthoughts. A cloud darted in front of the sun ten minutes before it was due to set.

34

And Then You Crash

The day before my chemo began, Stacey and I got drunk with Ron and Anna, Steve and Rita, on an excellent Pomerol of Ron's choice. It was the day that jihadists shot up the Paris offices of *Charlie Hebdo*, the satirical magazine. Also, a kosher market.

On steroids, given to combat the nausea that the chemicals cause, I became expansive, voluble. Unable to sleep, I stayed up until four in the morning writing and reading. It was a kind of euphoria. "Don't call it speed," the nurse said in a tone harsher than he probably intended. Nevertheless, I insist . . . chemotherapy means speeding on Thursday and Friday nights and then . . . then you crash. Nothing tastes good but you have to eat because the steroids make you hungry. The lemonade does not taste like lemonade. The ginger ale tastes like metal. Nothing tastes like itself.

On Wednesday night you begin taking the steroids. Five pills then, and five the next morning. You report to the hospital for your chemo on Thursday. After four hours hooked to an IV pole, plus two in the waiting room, they let you go home if you urinate a sufficient amount. They forbid you to take mass transit. They remind you to wear gloves at all times. You take a taxi home and more steroids. On Friday you return to the hospital and get a shot of Neulasta to bolster your immune system. More steroids. You go off the steroid regimen on Saturday night. By Sunday you are on the couch and from then until Wednesday afternoon you cannot get off your back. You have crashed.

35

Chemo

Nothing prepares you for chemo. If you're lucky you get the benefit of speed for a few hours. But then comes the fatigue, the numbness, the inability to get off the couch, the *disgust* you feel at the mention of food and nourishment.

You can't sleep.

You try to read great books (Proust, Tolstoy, Dostoyevsky, Stendhal, Balzac) but you can't focus.

You try to read your favorite spy and detective novels (Ambler, Chandler, Agatha Christie, Rex Stout) but you lose interest.

You watch the Knicks blow a ten-point lead in the fourth quarter.

You write caustic or clever letters to the editors of the *New York Review of Books* (protesting an apologist for a forgetful ex-Nazi), the *New York Times* (defending bow ties as a sartorial accessory), the *Wall Street Journal* (correcting a statement about the importance of Allied casualties in World War II), *Sports Illustrated* (remembering Howard Cosell), and *The Nation* (in which the tagline of an article about "Woody and Dylan" made you think of Woody Guthrie and Bob Dylan rather than about Woody Allen and Dylan Farrow).

By writing these letters you are asserting yourself, saying I am still alive don't count me out.

You quote Flaubert from your Commonplace Book: "Saint-Just was a theorist, who cared only about the masses, but showed no mercy for the individuals."

You stop watching the Knicks.

You sleep.

You get stoned.

One day you are living in a secret place somewhere north by northeast of London working for Allied intelligence, enduring difficult training sessions, experimenting and being experimented on. You have a wound. There are practical exercises and competitions, like marine boot camp but with intellectual variations, such as having to learn a language in one week, memorize the periodic table, and cheat at poker.

You read about wounds. Jacob wrestling with the angel, emerging with a lifelong limp and a blessed new name. Blind Milton, deaf Beethoven. Edmund Wilson's "The Wound and the Bow." Auden's "Letter to a Wound." You wonder whether you will ever be able to write something on that model.

You still can't sleep.

You watch too much television and hate yourself.

You catch your wife sobbing at her desk and you hate yourself.

You become a news junkie until you can't stand it anymore and you switch off the set.

You hate anchorman jargon: the "moral high ground," a "slippery slope," "the devil in the details," "the optics."

You and your wife watch *The Best Years of Our Lives* and choke up during the last scene, when Homer and Wilma marry and Teresa Wright and Dana Andrews embrace, pledging their troth.

You sleep.

The sweetest moment of the night is when you wake up sweating under the covers.

You observe the studied blandness, the smiles, the helpfulness while secretly the doctors and nurses and technicians are thinking, "We are trying out Gitmo tortures on you."

You swing from boredom to belligerence.

You rant against jeans that are fashionably ripped above the knees—as if to furnish irrefutable sartorial proof that "privilege" is bad. Didn't they used to call that slumming?

You imitate Joseph Cotten as an infirm geezer in a wheelchair craving a cigar in a rest home in *Citizen Kane*: "What a tiresome old man I have become."

You deliver an impromptu excoriation on the slow but steady decay of cultural values. What have they done to the English language? What happened to honor, dignity, charm, and truthfulness as virtues?

You repeat yourself, less effectively each time.

You write your autobiography but it is not the authorized version. A lot of it is fake.

You tell people you don't miss the taste, you miss the effect, of the martinis you are not allowed to drink. They would taste like iron filings.

You walk to the local liquor store for recreation and return with bottles of gin and single-malt scotch—bottles you will not drink, but touching them will (you hope) give you a contact high.

You take out your notebook and write: *Everything is either unreal or a bad deal, and everyone is invisible.* The electronic devices that people use have rendered them invisible. As an inveterate magazine junkie, you know that *Life* is dead and *Time* is unreal—either that or it's not really *Time*. It's a simulacrum, to use the approved academic word, itself a fake. Fake and unreal. Delusions, contradictions. Competitive yoga at Equinox.

Then the thought occurs to you: *I am the one who is unreal. I come from a different century, and I miss it, bloody though it was.*

You stand up too fast and you get dizzy.

You don't want to leave the apartment. You want visitors, but once they arrive you can't wait for them to leave. You hate yourself.

It will never be different. It will always be like this. It is like a snowstorm in Clinton, New York, where Hamilton College is—Clinton, "the Versailles of Utica," as the professor of theater, an aging dandy, put it, folding his hands. It is snowing horizontally. I am not the first person to say so. I am the black swan in the whiteness of February. The snow has whitewashed the truth. The snow has cleansed the dictator's teeth. I walk up the hill in the snow. I get as far as the gazebo before turning back in the snow. The snow has covered the ground. The land is whiter than the white wash of a white woman using powdered white detergent. It has always been snowing. It has never stopped snowing.

36

Roid Rage

For the first month I was cheerful, almost buoyant. I subscribe to a lot of magazines and brought them in to distribute among my fellow chemo patients and the nurses. And mostly I kept my cool. Mostly.

In the taxi from hospital to home one evening following a long day in the chemo suite, I fill Stacey in on the latest gossip about Paula and Zack, a couple we're obliged to spend time with, neither of whom has phoned or written to inquire about my treatment. It's raining and the lingering odor of the cabdriver's lunch and a surreptitious cigarette have made me slightly queasy. Chemo has heightened my sense of smell.

"Well," Stacey says. "That's Paula. What do you expect?"

"That's her all right. And him too. I never liked him. I don't like the way he treats her."

"Don't get upset," Stacey says.

"I'm *not* upset."

"Take it easy."

"Don't you think she should have phoned me by now?"

"Yes, but that's not the point."

"It is precisely the goddamn point."

"Lower your voice. She's just being who she is."

We stop at a traffic light. The driver looks at me in his rearview mirror then looks over his shoulder at Stacey. It is raining hard, windy too. A pedestrian loses the battle with his cheap umbrella.

"That's the kind of bullshit excuse for umbrellas that they make for suckers," I snarl. The only other sound is that of the windshield wipers.

"Why can't you just agree with me, damn it?"

"I do agree with you."

"Then why didn't you say so? Just say it."

"I did say so. And don't speak to me like that. I don't deserve it."

"No, you don't, but . . ."

"Don't get upset," Stacey repeats.

"I'm not upset."

"Stop or I'll get out of the cab."

"Okay, okay." I lower my voice.

We ride for a few minutes in silence. Stacey keeps her head turned away.

"But why shouldn't I get upset? Tell me that!

"And I hate the graham crackers they shove down my throat."

37

Under the Garden

I love first lines. The opening of Graham Greene's story "Under
the Garden," for example:

> It was only when the doctor said to him, "Of course the fact that you
> don't smoke is in your favour," Wilditch realized what it was he had
> been trying to convey with such tact. Dr Cave had lined up along one
> wall a series of X-ray photographs, the whorls of which reminded the
> patient of those pictures of the earth's surface taken from a great height
> that he had pored over at one period during the war, trying to detect the
> tiny grey seed of a launching ramp.

With the indirection that passes for a physician's professional
"tact," the opening sentence reveals that Wilditch, the protago-
nist, has just been handed a death sentence. The paragraph dwells
on the doctor's discomfort with speaking the bald truth ("what
it was he had been trying to convey"), his determination to skirt
the subject, with the result that the bitter prognostication of the
man's demise dawns on the reader in the same way that it dawns
on Wilditch: belatedly, like the answer to a riddle or trick question.

The names (Wilditch, Dr. Cave) may seem allegorical, but that
is perhaps as it should be in a piece of dreamlike fiction that sets
store (we learn later) by "the power of the name." Wilditch does

have an untamed side, and in the extended sequence that gives the story its title, he is a little boy lost in a cave under the garden behind the house in which he grew up.

The simile in the second sentence is sublimely on the mark, the X-ray likened to aerial photography of enemy territory "during the war"—the war that need not be named because it was the central event of the entire century. The diseased body is likened to a landscape, and a war-torn zone at that, dominated by destructive weapons and therefore a likely target of destruction itself. It is a brilliant touch. The sentence conveys something about the medical profession—its appeal to the impersonal, the technical, the clinical and allegedly scientific—introducing at the same time a critical piece of information about the past life of our hero, now reduced pathetically to "the patient," like an accused man standing powerless before a tribunal.

The word "trying" appears twice in this short paragraph—the first time in reference to the doctor's inadequate use of language, the second time in reference to Wilditch's work in the war. The word almost always implies failure or futility, and it hangs in the air here, perhaps to remind us that for all its air of precision, the medical profession is as approximate and as founded on guesswork as military maneuvers—ill-named "surgical strikes," for example—and that it is the inevitable fate of the human body to decline into a state of decay or rebellion, and when that happens, life becomes a terminal trial.

"Under the Garden" is much the longest story in Greene's 1963 collection, which he called *A Sense of Reality*. It is a shrewd composite title for a book of stories that lives up to an ideal that Coleridge described in *Biographia Literaria* (chapter 14). Coleridge, accounting for his contribution to the *Lyrical Ballads*, tells us he aimed at writing poems in which "the incidents and agents were to be, in part at least, supernatural" and nevertheless felt "real." "And,"

Coleridge adds, "real in this sense they have been to every human being who, from whatever source of delusion, has at any time believed himself under supernatural agency."

Not until the last paragraph of "Under the Garden" do we encounter the word "cancer," and then only once.

38

The End

The day Graham Greene died
I didn't know he had died
but months earlier I'd written
a poem and called it "The End
of the Affair" stealing his title
and on this April day in 1991
I went to the Blue Fox bookstore
which no longer exists
on Aurora Street in Ithaca
and bought *The End of the Affair*
thinking it was time I read it
and I started reading it right away
it was great he really knew adultery
and I still remember the surprise
when you find out whom Bendrix
loses Sarah to, the one rival
he could never hope to vanquish,
the God who answered her prayer
I stayed up all night reading
reached the end and the next day
on the radio he died

39

Falling in Love Again

Then he fell in love. It ended badly. Her name was Reba or Amy or Beth. Lust ran on parallel tracks: Andrea, Susan, and Laurie. It was a very good year. Laurie's father drove them home from the tryst. In the kitchen with the window open he sat with his hair wet and did his algebra homework listening to the Rangers game on the radio. Then he wrote: Love's the boy with the brilliant brain who commits petty crimes to see if he can get away with them until he meets a girl who thinks she understands his wounded self. Love is a debt without a maturity date, an unequal equation, a black market drug you have to pay for in cash in the backseat of a taxi driven by a thug in the employ of a mob boss. Love is deaf. Love is death. Love is the wound that will never heal. Love is Laurie, love is fear of getting involved with Laurie, he wonders where she is today. Love is an imp with a toy sword that turns into a real sword in a horror movie. Love is the offspring of the goddess of biology, whom the Greeks called Aphrodite. Love is the son of maidenly beauty, who made love to passionate Psyche at night when she could not see him, and only then. Love is the wine that tastes better than even joy's grape to Keats in the throes of the nightingale's song.

But then—Who had stopped loving whom? Had changed? Was running away? Did it matter? He remembered his pleasure when he let himself into her flat the first time, fixed himself a drink, sipped it, got into her bed, and waited for her there, knowing she would come. Now everything was wrong. He was a slob in her bathtub, spilled his seed on her pristine sheets, and was always late because of her, who used too much eye shadow and blush. Her face looked as garish as her voice turned shrill.

So they fought and made love. Then they stopped fighting. Then they stopped making love. In public they acted married. Not enough lime in the daiquiris he made, and the salsa could have used more jalapeño peppers. She was constipated every weekend she spent with him, and it was his fault. She was a hardworking Virgo, and he craved a cigarette, feeling like an outlaw. You could tell he loved her by the way he ranted about her.

40

Nothingness

I write poems. I like writing poems. It doesn't matter if anyone wants to read them.

But today—today I am a French novelist. The first word I type is *néant*—nothingness. That is as far as I get.

It is better in French.

This is how I solved the problem: I went through a short story (Mary McCarthy's "Man in the Brooks Brothers Shirt") sentence by sentence, and wherever a noun appeared, I substituted the word "nothing."

Nothing happened.

The result was a conceptual work inasmuch as the idea preceded and determined the content.

I applied the technique to Jean-Paul Sartre's *Nausea* on a day I felt nauseated but that is just one possibility.

There is, the novelist said, "a difference between fantasy and fiction." But he didn't say what it was. My book on nothing has come to nothing, but I watched Olivier's *Hamlet* last night, and where were Rosencrantz and Guildenstern, and what happened to some of the big speeches, "what's Hecuba to him" and "what a piece of work is a man," for example? But he did read his lines beautifully. How often Hamlet says things thrice. Words, words, words. Well, well, well. Except my life, except my life, except my life.

41

Syllabus

Most of the patients here are men, here being the Sidney Kimmel Center for Prostate and Urologic Cancers. Prostate, bladder, testicular: unlike the unisex bladder, the other two are male cancers, the latter most likely to afflict young men under forty. Those around me are mostly over fifty, pale, and out of shape. The young men wear knit caps pulled low on their foreheads, trying to look like just another Brooklyn hipster; the older men don't care if their chemo-baldness shows. I don't see myself in them but that's the power of denial, and it's a good thing. Some of the patients are accompanied by one or two friends who try to make light of the situation by talking about sports while their friend sits, stone-faced, tethered to a steady drip. Sometimes entire families crowd into one cubicle, where there's room for one guest to sit while the others stand.

But usually it's mothers or wives with their husbands or sons. The women fuss while the patient sleeps. They read outdated women's magazines, or knit, or embroider. Stacey brings her laptop and works or watches a movie. Once, a female patient nearby had a panic attack, something my nurse said might happen to me. "When we give you this drug for the first time," he said, "you might feel as if you're going to die. It will seem real to you. I'm not kidding." I didn't say anything. "Don't worry," he said. "It doesn't happen very often and we know what to do when it does."

My friend Jane, who did her graduate work in music history, comes to keep me company one Thursday when I am receiving the poisons in my port. A former cancer patient herself, Jane is one of the few friends I have welcomed to sit with me during treatment. Stacey needs a break, and after dropping me off and waiting to make sure that Jane will keep our date, she's gone to visit a museum with a friend. Jane knows the drill. She'll understand if I doze off. She'll bring me water and won't make demands. Jane is writing a book about movie music, and if all goes well we are going to talk about Elmer Bernstein's march in *The Great Escape* and Jerry Fielding's soundtrack for *The Wild Bunch*. Jane's daughter, home for the holidays, told her she signed up for a course on Shakespeare's tragedies. But—Jane sighed—the other courses were beginning yoga, "Disney Princesses," "Derrida's Politics," and wine and beer tasting (pass-fail). We laughed.

I have had to take a leave and so I am not teaching the course I love to teach, "Literature and Ideas of the West" at the New School. The course begins with Genesis and *The Odyssey*, Erich Auerbach's essay on an episode in each, poems by Marvell ("The Garden") and Tennyson ("Ulysses"), a Kafka parable ("Abraham"), a short story by Henry James ("The Tree of Knowledge") and one by Katherine Mansfield ("Bliss"), and three more "blissful" poems: Thomas Gray's "Ode on a Distant Prospect of Eton College" ("where ignorance is bliss, / 'Tis folly to be wise"), Wordsworth's "Daffodils" ("the bliss of solitude"), and Elizabeth Bishop's "Crusoe in England" ("the bliss of what?"). Next we read the book of Jonah and "The Rime of the Ancient Mariner"; Byron lampooning Homer in canto two of *Don Juan*, and Kierkegaard's attempt to fathom Abraham in *Fear and Trembling*; Oedipus and Antigone;

Hamlet on the fence, and Freud analyzing him and rejecting both the Judeo-Christian and Greco-Roman worldviews. Then Nietzsche, Freud on the uncanny, with readings in Poe, Graham Greene, May Sinclair, Borges, Shirley Jackson, Sholem Aleichem et al., *1984* compared to *Brave New World.* The prose of persuasion (Virginia Woolf's *A Room of One's Own*) and narration (three Hemingway stories and Gertrude Stein's *Autobiography of Alice B. Toklas*). Midcentury America: Richard Yates's *Revolutionary Road*, James Baldwin's *Notes of a Native Son.* Susan Sontag's *Illness as Metaphor* paired with Kafka's "Hunger Artist." Finally, the book of Ruth, Keats's "Ode to a Nightingale," and two of Somerset Maugham's stories, "The Alien Corn" and "The Lotus Eater."

Like the anthology, it is an unsung art form: the syllabus.

42

Commencement Speech

Good news at the hospital: "The discomfort you are feeling is normative." Everyone on chemo is entitled to at least one all-out rant, and here's your chance. You can yell at the staff or call your (male) boss a pussy in front of witnesses. You can fire someone or write someone out of your will or punch a hole in the kitchen cupboard. You can phone a fool you've put up with and tell him what you really think. You may send an e-mail you will come to regret someday but someday isn't now. You can throw a paranoid fit. It's *normative.*

You can speechify to your heart's content, waxing nostalgic for the week in April 1968 when the spirit of revolution prevailed at Columbia University, but then you risk sounding like the high school quarterback or prom queen, who peaked when they were seventeen. Some of my classmates, many of them coreligionists, waited for the revolution as hopefully as their great-grandparents had waited for the Messiah and redemption. I know someone in this category to whom I feel like saying, "Johnny, my friend, you never were very bright. But I love you anyway."

You can discern the shadow of fascism in the rise of one presidential candidate and the specter of socialism in another. You can lament the fate of Venezuela and the misery Chávez and his cronies made for the masses. You can deplore the return of anti-Semitism, which is to history what the speed of light is to Einstein's theory of relativity: the one constant. You can address uncertainty, not Heisenberg's, though that, too, but Wall Street's worry, and perhaps invoke as an example the Brexit movement in England, but first be sure to explain what Brexit is, because nobody here knows.

Or you may devote your speech to the original transgression in Genesis, chapter 3. Why was the one proscribed act that of eating a fruit from the tree of knowledge? Why eating rather than walking behind a certain bush or swimming in the pond or examining the genitalia of a tulip? Why a fruit? Had the Lord been Greek he might have said: You may look at anything but your face reflected in the pond. But the Lord being Hebrew specifies that it is a fruit, sweet and crisp, whose mortal taste brought death into the world. It is a fruit that opens your eyes. You eat it and gain knowledge and lose your innocence, but it is curious, is it not, that the knowledge you gain will be carnal and the imperative you obey will be to be fruitful and multiply. Walter Kirn has propounded the theory that the expulsion of Adam and Eve was the world's first drug bust, a clever conceit. But an unanswerable question remains: Why did a fruit from a tree embody original sin? And why was knowledge outlawed, not action or experience, deceit or treachery, violence or greed?

The next week's hellfire sermon might commence with the observation that by chapter 4 of Genesis we have our first murder mystery, a fratricide, with a victim, a culprit, a motive, and an unerring detective.

43

The Exquisite Corpse

Finally I've come up with the motive for the murder in the detective novel I am writing in my sleep. It's called *The Exquisite Corpse*. Helen Highwater, the character vaguely modeled on Madonna, kills Roberta Esperanto, the character vaguely modeled on Lady Gaga. In her hotel room bathtub. During a showbiz convention in Los Angeles where recent Oscar winners and other major celebrities will entertain an audience that includes Bill and Hillary Clinton. The motive? Lady Gaga has unearthed some of the facts about Madonna that she had labored to keep secret: that, for example, she is a Republican. Of course these characters are really based on poetry world personalities, but I can't say who is who without serious repercussions, and I have changed the sex of half the characters so they probably won't recognize themselves.

44

The Editorial "We"

The letters to the editor in newspapers and magazines, many of which start with "As," are consistently entertaining. As a professional entomologist I must take issue with the statement that flies are attracted not to vinegar but to honey. On the contrary, honey attracts wasps and ants (Hymenoptera), while many flies (Diptera) are drawn to vinegar as a moth is drawn to a flame. As a portfolio manager whose superior investment profitability is based on correct fact finding, I am offended by the statement that men are better than women at Scrabble, because neither sex has a genetic advantage in nailing down facts and correcting errors, which your writer alleges to be the key to winning at Scrabble, which, may I remind you, is a game, and games are not life. As the fifth-generation owner of Katz's Delicatessen on the Lower East Side I am deeply saddened to witness the disappearance of a fellow culinary landmark, the Carnegie Deli. As a convicted felon who plans to pursue a degree in higher education upon his release from the Coxsackie Correctional Facility I appreciated the visiting poet and am grateful for the gift subscription. As a Mets fan I am still outraged that the team traded Tom Seaver for what Ira Gershwin would call "plenty o' nuttin'" and the fact that this happened thirty-eight years ago does nothing to lessen my indignation.* As an animal rights activist, a reformed male chauvinist, a working mother, a woman who happens not to be a mom and feels left out when it is assumed that all women are moms or should be. As a Canadian. As a confessed sex addict who teaches a course on "genre and gender." As a former public defender who worries about the tendency to romanticize jailhouse lawyers. As a sports psychology consultant, a season ticket holder, a football widow, an executive worried about the decline of attendance at baseball games. As a realist, a neo-Keynesian, a revisionist, an opponent of intersectionality brainwashing. A Kennedy-era liberal. A woman of a certain age.

Your credentials are in order, ladies and gentlemen. None of you inhaled or had sex with "that woman," and nobody declared "mission accomplished" like a premature ejaculation. You are who you say you are, all of you, though each is subject to the impostor complex, the nightmare in which everyone finds out you're a fake, you never completed that last course in French or physics and you will not graduate. Everyone sees through you.

And all of these correspondents are versions of me.

---

* In return for Seaver, the Mets received Pat Zachry, Doug Flynn, Steve Henderson, and Dan Norman. Unconscionable.

45

Oblivion

The voice asks: Will I die? Never aloud, even to Stacey. I lie in bed and imagine the world without me.

Of course, there are practical things to attend to—time-consuming papers, financial statements, legal documents, business affairs. How best to take care of my wife and my son. That's the easy part.

More difficult it is to ponder the absence of myself from the world. How short is our collective memory: I think of gaudy poets dead and now nearly forgotten by all but a handful of PhD candidates. How swiftly the absence swallows us. The "forgotten man" that FDR remembered in his dynamic first term is overlooked because he is one of the powerless many, because there is nothing distinctive about him, and because, as Jesus says, the poor we shall always have with us. But the beloved absent friend is forgotten simply because he or she has disappeared.

The concept of my absence defeats all philosophy. I cannot grasp it. Oblivion: I thought I understood it pretty well when I read Dickinson and Frost. But the deaths of friends feel more like disappearances than deaths. In the old days, before I got sick, I might, if lucky, run into the ghost of one or another pal as I walked in a familiar garden or park—and sometimes I still view the familiar features of a friend of long standing, though usually from a distance, with no chance to have a conversation with her or him. And I wonder whether there will be some who will feel my ghostly presence after I've gone, and for how long.

It keeps me awake some nights—oblivion—the end of consciousness—impossible to conceive, though each time they give me a general anesthetic I learn a little more about the way it works. There is this to be said about general anesthesia: it lessens the fear of death.

46

Dostoyevsky

Bar stools have this much in common with the chemotherapy waiting room. They're full of bullshit artists and compulsive story-of-my-life big mouths. Downstairs at the Otto bar, the man next to me tells us his life story. What set him off was the copy of *The Odyssey* (trans. Robert Fitzgerald) that I was reading. I forget the logic. He talked nonstop for ninety minutes. Then he gave me his card. It said he was a psychotherapist. He said he went into that field because he's "a good listener."

In the waiting room, Dostoyevsky shows up and delivers an awesome speech in which the phrase "they haven't suffered enough" is repeated. They, the enemies of humanity, are everywhere. Their wives don't love them, their husbands cheat on them, they have no balls (men) or tits (women), they have that scared look of patients entering a hospital knowing they will die there and yet I tell you *they haven't suffered enough!* Their souls are still at the first corridor of limbo. Their evil is an illness as well as a sin and their souls are not ready for the first treatment, the first hellfire sermon. *They haven't suffered enough!* They don't know the meaning of suffering, because they lack the education that only the experience of failure and defeat can give them. *They haven't suffered enough!* They will never know the meaning of life. Though you tell me they have suffered—in their bodies, and in their minds, and because of their hateful ungrateful siblings, and their spiteful ex-spouses, and their whining brats, and their phony colleagues, their confederates in falsehood, their treacherous friends, it isn't enough—I tell you it's a pity but *they haven't suffered enough!*

47

The Spiritual Connection

No writer has ever known my soul as well as Dostoyevsky did when I was twenty-three years old. Our spiritual connection lasted decades but reached its zenith in a six-month period in 1972 that began in Paris where I read *The Gambler* and *Crime and Punishment* in a Left Bank garret and continued in Cambridge where, under the guidance of my philosopher friend Robert Allen, I read *The Brothers Karamazov*. Dostoyevsky burned like a candle in my Cambridge digs on Chesterton Road when the coal miners went on strike and we had brownouts every night. We called him Dusty.

In *Aspects of the Novel* E. M. Forster compares a passage in George Eliot's *Adam Bede* to one in *The Brothers Karamazov* and concludes with a sigh that Eliot was a preacher while Dostoyevsky was a prophet. The comparison is beautifully made and Forster is right. But a prophet can sound like a monomaniac, perhaps especially if he is as great a scoundrel as was Dostoyevsky. A compulsive gambler, utterly devoid of self-control, he would shamelessly beg for funds that he would squander at the tables in Baden-Baden or Wiesbaden, the "Roulettenberg" of *The Gambler*. Somerset Maugham, who loved Dostoyevsky's novels, wrote that he could think of no one in whom the discrepancy between the man and his works was greater. Dostoyevsky was, in Maugham's words, "vain, envious, quarrelsome, suspicious, cringing, selfish, boastful, unreliable, inconsiderate, narrow and intolerant." There were no depths of self-abasement to which this "odious character" would not descend. Perhaps this is partly why with Dostoyevsky, as with Hemingway, the ideal age at which to read his books is before you are twenty-five years old. After you are thirty some of the most divinely inspired fiction in world literature has an inadvertent element of comedy if only because the questions that animate the prophet—"Why are people poor? Why is the babe poor? Why is the steppe barren? Why don't they hug each other and kiss? Why don't they sing songs of joy? Why are they so dark from black misery? Why don't they feed the babe?"—lose their immediacy when you reach the age at which you can no longer decide on a whim to pack a suitcase and fly to Paris for an undefined period of time.

Dostoyevsky wrote his masterpieces in a great hurry, and only as a last resort, to erase his gambling debts. He was the son of a murder victim, dispatched by his serfs, which is in line with Freud's analysis of Dostoyevsky and parricide. He suffered from epileptic fits (see *The Idiot*) and was, in sum, basically a jerk with genius who survived an awe-inspiring ordeal. On April 23, 1849, at the age of twenty-seven, Dostoyevsky was arrested for belonging to a group of crazy liberal loudmouth intellectuals. Sentenced to be executed, he faced a firing squad in the freezing rain. But it turned out to be a mock execution and Dostoyevsky went back to his cell the shape and size of a coffin convinced that it is better and wiser to be a saintly fool in Siberia than to be a pimp in St. Petersburg. Released in 1854, he dashed off *Crime and Punishment*.

On November 11, 1918—three years shy of Dusty's centenary birthday—World War I ended, and in graveyards in the Ukraine and Byelorussia, in Latvia and Estonia, the ghosts of schoolchildren in tatters took time off from the Russian Revolution and gathered together in public spaces to shout "Hurrah for Karamazov!"

48

"Myself, When Stoned"

Why I write: George Orwell has an essay with this title and it's to his credit that he gives a straight answer. He has a political purpose: he is "against totalitarianism and for democratic socialism." He wants to change the world and thinks that it can be done. My ambitions are more modest. I write to assert my will to live. To prove I exist. When all I want to do is sleep, I make myself write. I love writing, have long championed the practice of daily writing, and will not stop now. Even on days of maximum fatigue, apathy, and disgust, I need to spend an hour at the computer. If I do nothing more than rephrase a thought in yesterday's paragraphs, I have done something. And if I add a single sentence, it's a victory. Should I date the entries? No, just number them. You can always shuffle the order and add titles later.

These are the two misprints on telegrams or envelopes that have given me the most pleasure: "Lionet Trifling" and "John Ashberg." Nor is it a coincidence that the two men thus designated have exerted the greatest influence on my mind and my art. Ashbery will turn up in these pages sooner or later as himself, or as JA, after his early poem "The Picture of Little J. A. in a Prospect of Flowers." As for Trilling, my time in graduate school at Columbia was pretty much a bust except for the year I worked as his research assistant.

Trilling, who cross-examined "the liberal imagination" as much as he may be said to have advocated it, was the legendary Columbia professor Allen Ginsberg called at one in the morning from the West End Bar to say he was in trouble again or had seen God.

I loved the subtlety of Trilling's intelligence as it manifested itself in a prose of complexity, ambivalence, and difficulty, three conditions of mind that he valued. His prose style, characterized by its subordinate clauses, reversals, and qualifications, captured a supple mind in motion. In his office, I got to ask him about the New York intellectuals and the Alger Hiss case and Delmore Schwartz and contemporary poetry (which he distrusted because "the poets are always giving each other prizes"), and Allen Ginsberg (who was *not* the inspiration for Tertan in "Of This Time, of That Place," the best of Trilling's short stories), and Baudelaire's "artificial paradise" and psychedelic drugs and the perilous tendency of the time to consider madness a virtue, a concomitant of genius. When I brought my mother to meet him, Trilling treated her with unforced graciousness and evinced not an iota of condescension. Detractors questioned his genuineness. But I never doubted it. Merely in conducting himself as he did, he taught me more "than all the sages can," to borrow a line from Wordsworth, Trilling's favorite poet.

Trilling and Ashbery: moral seriousness on the one side and homosexual aestheticism on the other. Susan Sontag nailed it: "The two pioneering forces of modern sensibility are Jewish moral seriousness and homosexual aestheticism and irony."

Against the pressures of reality, the imagination presses back (Wallace Stevens). From ominous circumstance, outrageous fortune, the aesthetic way proposes itself as an escape.

"Myself, When Stoned": a brilliant title. Dear JA: Did you ever write it?

Hours have gone by since I wrote that sentence after crossing out two paragraphs devoted to the question of what the Martian whose existence Noam Chomsky postulates would, if asked to hazard an opinion based strictly on TV commercials, say about the human species.

The life of the party does not like it when he finds out what people are saying behind his back in the sobriety of a weekday morning.

Oh, my head. So this is what it's like to have a hangover. For all the drinking I've done, I never had to pay that particular price. Whenever I drank to excess, I always made sure to drink a quart of grapefruit juice or lemonade and take three Advil before going to bed. I never woke up with a hangover. It took chemotherapy to teach me how it feels to have a hangover. Lesson learned. Those nights when I drank three or four martinis, each one a triple, how did I manage to get home safely?

The blood transfusion I had yesterday was, just for the record, the third in three months. Blood pressure: 116 over 70. Pulse: 93. Temperature: 97. Normal.

49

Bloomsday

At the end of the necessary four months of chemo, the oncologist beamed as if I had scored an A+ on the final. He held the scan results. "We're clearing you for the operation," he said. Everyone looked happy. It meant that upon graduation I could take a month off before I went on to the next step, the five-hour surgery in which they remove your bladder, some lymph nodes, and choice other parts of you and reorganize your insides while you are deeply under a general anesthetic.

We picked June 16 for the operation, Bloomsday, the day in 1904 when James Joyce first courted Nora Barnacle, a chambermaid from Galway City—the day in Dublin that he spent eight years memorializing in *Ulysses*, the definitive monument of modernism. This was my daily poem on June 16, 1996. I was teaching at Bennington College and I wrote it in the pocket notebook that I am rarely without:

It's Bloomsday in Dublin
and wherever Ulysses works
as an advertising man
with an unfaithful wife
as I sit here listening
to a lecture on Flannery

O'Connor, Frank O'Connor,
and the O'Hara boys, John
and Frank, I think of going
to Dublin with you buying
a toy wedding ring at
Woolworth's and the phrase
"mock funeral" comes
to me I don't know what it
means though I remember being
the groom at a mock wedding
with a girl named Ann in 1956
I was eight and so was she
and all the other children
were in the procession it was
the first hot night in June and
yes she said yes I will Yes

On June 15 I write to a friend, "Chemo was so infernal it makes
me feel grateful just to be alive now that the terrible side effects—
some of them anyway—have begun to recede. My hair is growing
back, my appetite has returned, I'm no longer as fatigued as I was,
and my reward is . . . tomorrow's operation."

50

Tom Collins

He woke up dry. The nurse said he could apply the waterlogged sponge to his lips but was not allowed to drink anything. He motioned to her to come near. In her ear he whispered conspiratorially that what he really wanted was a Tom Collins. He hadn't had a Tom Collins in maybe thirty years. But he wanted one now. He thought of the tall frosty Collins glass full of ice cubes and fizz in 1965, the summer of the riots in Watts, floral frocks and folk songs. He drank a Collins nightly, usually a rum Collins, sometimes a vodka Collins, at the rustic bowling alley and cocktail lounge in Rhinebeck where he and Norman schmoozed while the Dorsey band on the jukebox played "Marie." And then by the miracle of morphine, there he was, with his co-counselors at Camp Harrow in the Catskills: hipster Norman, fun-loving Milty, brilliant though homely Lillian, Joan the sophisticate, and nature boy Abe.

"Hey, champ." Norman calls his close friends "champ."

"Norman," I say. "What are you doing here?"

As nonchalant as the half-shade sunglasses he sports indoors Norman is my guru, two years older than I, infinitely wiser and better informed. Through his tutelage I understood that my opposition to the war in Vietnam, which dated back to LBJ's escalation of the conflict, was consonant with such cultural developments

as the freewheeling Bob Dylan, Phil Ochs, Leadbelly, "signifying
monkey," Paul Krassner and *The Realist* magazine, and the Gas-
light Café on MacDougal Street.

In work shirt and jeans Norman is all smiles. "Nice catch."

"I was lucky."

"That ball was a screaming line drive."

"It came straight at me. I didn't have time to think."

A mediocre athlete, I did have that one moment of glory best ex-
pressed in a display of false modesty, for when the counselors de-
feated the waiters 5–4 while the campers watched in August 1965,
my catch ended the game in our favor.

I tell Norman I finished *The Old Man and the Sea.*

"What did you think?"

"It was a little shallow," I say, an unwitting pun that wins me
points.

Norman and I have to write the songs and skits for the gray dev-
ils versus the blue angels—or was it the gray swordsmen versus the
blue scribes?—in color war.

"For the march," he says, "I think we should use 'Alexander's
Ragtime Band' and for the cheer a calypso."

At the social tonight I'm going to dance with Nadine.

On the backs of envelopes of letters sent home (as required,
twice weekly) some of the girls write "God bless the U.S. Male"
or "Deliver de-letter de-sooner de-better." Everyone feels solemn
when the flag is lowered and "Taps" is played. And at evening's end
the girls will sing "Save Your Heart for Me" with sweet sincerity.

51

The Admissions Officer

Home is New York City, where the homeless are at home, and even the rich can understand the homeless as an existential condition if not as an objective reality.

You're that rare thing, a native New Yorker, the Yale admissions officer said.

Yes, I've lived in the city all my life except one summer in Canada.

What's your favorite place in the city?

My friends and I call it the campus. It's the last sloping lawn on the upper level of Fort Tryon Park near the exit leading to Fort Washington Avenue and Cabrini Boulevard. It's an easy walk from the Cloisters museum where I sometimes go to look at the Unicorn Tapestries and Robert Campin's Mérode triptych. When you leave the museum, you walk south and follow a winding path and you reach this sloping lawn. It's just a lawn with a paved path around it and a three-foot stone wall facing the Hudson River. You can see the George Washington Bridge from the campus. It's just to our south, big as life. Stand *there*, turn left, and there it is. On warm days in June and August, people bring blankets and books—Shakespeare's sonnets, a psychology textbook—and read them on the lawn, as on a college campus. There are flower gardens nearby, row upon row of colorful flowers in tiers with walking paths separating them. Near the exit there's a homely sign with these words in italic script: "Let no one say, and say it to your shame, that all was beauty here, until you came."

Mr. Oliver, the admissions officer conducting the interview, wore a brown-checked tweed suit with cuffs on the trousers, a light-blue Oxford button-down shirt, a thin solid-red silk knit tie, and shiny brown wingtips. I wore the olive-colored three-piece wool suit I had bought at Barney's for just this occasion, and not until this minute do I make the connection between the color of my suit and the name of the admissions officer. My father, in his gray Brooks Brothers business suit with navy-blue tie and white shirt with spread collar, waited in an adjacent room. After quizzing me to make sure that I really did read the *Times* every day, Mr. Oliver asked me about Hannah Arendt because in my application I boasted about winning a synagogue debate in which I had defended her book on Eichmann and her "banality of evil" argument. Mr. Oliver also wondered why I spelled God "G—d," which is what Lubavitchers do unto this day and which I didn't stop doing until college. Then he asked, "Are you a Kennedy man?"

This was in October 1965.

I said that I liked Bobby, who was then the junior senator from New York, but am disappointed that he hasn't come out more strongly against the Vietnam War.

"So you oppose the war in Vietnam?"

"Vehemently."

My father asked Mr. Oliver what my chances were. Mr. Oliver smiled noncommittally, but when he thought I was out of earshot he said in a low voice, "You can be proud of your boy." I pretended not to hear but felt pretty good, because I wasn't going to be hearing any such compliments from my dad, who was always very decent to me, very encouraging, but held the elders' view that praise of one's progeny should be withheld lest the offspring develop a swelled head.

My father visited the library while I sat in on Paul Weiss's class in metaphysics, the most memorable moment of which came when the professor, summarizing an epistemological argument, spoke of two Japanese Buddhist monks on a bridge, one of whom says, "The fish below are happier than we are," and the other retorts, "How can you know, not being a fish?" and the first monk gets the last word: "How can you know what I know, not being me?" The students chuckled, then returned to what they were really avid to argue: whether a preemptive attack on Nazi Germany would have been justified in 1939, though this question had no discernible relation to the course's syllabus or to the Zen of ichthyology.

Afterward my father and I linked up at the Beinecke Library, Yale's great new rare books library, and we walked back to the car. I could hardly contain my enthusiasm.

"What did he ask you?" my father asked, it being understood that "he" was the admissions officer who interviewed me.

"He asked me about Kennedy and Vietnam," I said, and gave him a recap of the entire exchange.

"Don't ever tell anyone your politics," my father said. It was not the first time he had warned me. It was his firm belief that politics and religion are strictly off-limits in polite company and that reticence on the subjects was in order when you went to a job interview. "Never let anyone know what you're thinking," he liked to say.

Good advice. But I was lucky. Two days later a full-page ad appeared in the *New York Times*. It was a petition to end the war in Vietnam and included dozens of Yale professors' names including that of Richard Oliver.

That day, driving with my father on the Merritt Parkway, with the spectacular autumn foliage on both sides of us—I think we stopped to take it in and then went and enjoyed a filet of flounder dinner at some fancy restaurant—was one of the great days of my life.

"I can see myself at Yale," I told my father in the car.

"It's very expensive," my father said.

"I can get a loan and a Regents' scholarship."

"They won't let you use that outside of New York State."

I had to admit that was a strike against Yale. Still, I said, "I can get a job after school and take out a loan."

"If you went to City College we'd buy you a car of your own," my father said. City College was free.

"Mother told me," I said. I didn't want a car. I wanted to go to Columbia.

"Did you hear about this special program they're developing at City College?"

"I read about it in the *Times* last week."

"*Nu?*"

"It's good to have a backup," I said. "I would still rather go to Columbia or Yale."

"So," he said as we reached the stop sign where Seaman Avenue empties into Dyckman Street, "you have your heart set on it?"

I nodded. "After all it was you who told me about the advantages of an Ivy League education."

This was true. My father admired venerable American institutions: Harvard and Yale, the New York Stock Exchange, Yankee Stadium, Brooks Brothers, *Showboat*; he loved America as only a refugee from Hitler's Germany, overjoyed at being spared, can love his adopted homeland. He also loved knowledge for its own sake. Some late nights I would arrive home to see him asleep in his favorite chair, legs up, with the *Encyclopedia Britannica* opened to an ancient battle (Marathon, Thermopylae), a master of gallows humor (Christian Morgenstern), the history of the Federal Reserve Board, fine points of Robert's Rules of Order, or the lives of Alexander, Leonardo, Galileo, Goethe, Disraeli, or Winston Churchill.

"All right," my father said, signifying that this would be his last word on the subject. As he turned left on Dyckman, right on Broadway, and left again on Arden Street, he said, "What did you think of the rabbi's sermon last Shabbos?"

52

Columbia

So I went to an Ivy League college—not Yale, though I did make it to the waiting list, but Columbia, which was only twenty minutes away on the IRT, so I could live at home, at least for the first couple of years, a money-saving gesture my parents appreciated. And Columbia was where Lionel Trilling taught, and Mark Van Doren, too. Even I had heard of them. Also, I liked the image of myself wearing a blue blazer at a smoker in the lounge of one of the older Columbia dorms, Furnald or Hartley, where you could talk to the dean of the college as played by Fredric March. If my aim in life was to become a gentleman, Columbia was the ticket.

As a freshman I had Edward Said (pronounced "Sa-YEED") for a course in expository writing centering on the poetry of Donne, Coleridge, and Wallace Stevens. This was long before Said became famous as the author of *Orientalism*. Edward even had a silly nickname, in which a foreshortened version of his first name rhymed with his last ("Ed said"). My paper on Coleridge's "Dejection" ode won me an A, which was hard to get in those days, especially from Said, who was electrifying and altogether a pleasure except for the time he ridiculed Jim McMillian, maybe the greatest basketball player in Columbia's history, who sat next to me sometimes and on this occasion failed to answer satisfactorily a question about

John Donne's poem "The Canonization." The amiable McMillian, who went on to have a fruitful professional career with the Los Angeles Lakers, shrugged it off. In those days, after all, professors routinely reprimanded students who had shirked their homework.

Unlike a lot of other students, I looked straight, no beard or long hair, but like nearly everyone else on campus except economists and athletes, I subscribed to the prevailing climate of intellectual opinion, which can be inferred from the primary texts in my first-semester courses: we read *To the Finland Station,* Edmund Wilson's history of Marxism, in freshman English; in French we read the avatars of existentialism, Sartre, Camus, Ionesco, Simone de Beauvoir. You were supposed to be in favor of free love, sodomy, avant-garde art, and jeans, and alliteratively against the past, the parents, and the parietal hours.

What, you never heard of parietal hours? This was the era of *in loco parentis*—when universities were obliged to discharge the duties of parents, and wholesomeness was the expected norm. In those benighted times of daring panty raids, the student body at Columbia (and most of the other Ivy League colleges) was male.* In the dorms, toilets and shared shower rooms with minimal privacy were down the hall. A fellow could have a girl in his dorm room twice a month, on alternate Saturday evenings, from nine PM until midnight. You needed to keep the door to your room open the width of a book, a requirement modified by the wiseass who introduced the idea of using a book of matches. God help you if your date was still in your room at half past midnight. It was an

---

* Both Columbia, all boys, and Barnard, all girls, existed under the university's umbrella. Each had its own core curriculum and student activities center. Some upper-level Columbia courses welcomed Barnard students, and vice versa. But most of the mixing went on outside the classroom. Columbia remained all male until 1982.

infraction punishable by the University Dormitory Council, which consisted of righteous upperclassmen who took pride in strict enforcement of the dormitory regulations.

The one time I broke the rule, I was rooming with an alto saxophonist in a two-room walk-through suite in Hartley Hall. He, an Eric Dolphy enthusiast, was away at a jazz festival for the weekend. I had lucked into a Barnard girl as horny as I was, and we were making out when an alarm sounded and I knew it was one in the morning. We had taken off most of our clothes, but that was as far as it went, and I think we were secretly relieved to be interrupted. We got dressed quickly and I walked her back to her dorm feeling guilty and embarrassed and scared.

The UDC had not yet convened to decide on my penalty when, on the next Sunday evening, I returned to my dorm room after spending the weekend with my parents and found that my roommate's psychedelic peace and love posters had been ripped off the wall and torn in pieces. The guys across the hall, two of them football players whom I had tutored in economics and French, had forced their way in.

I knocked on their door and, for my trouble, got punched in the glasses, which flew across the room.

"But I tutored you in economics," I said lamely.

My adviser, a poetry-loving professor of government who had worked in the State Department when JFK was president, told me that if I were to say nothing about the incident, he'd see to it that the UDC would let me off the hook on the dormitory infraction. And so it went.

That was the year when a Barnard junior shacked up with a Columbia senior in an off-campus apartment, and the news made the front page of the *New York Times*. Suddenly the "we" of sociological construction came into being. We, the permissive offspring of a prosperous postwar generation, were on the cusp of amazing change—and were agents of that change. We who blew smoke rings from the last row of the lecture hall had revolutionary fever and were intent on celebrating the naked body in the mud of an ecstatic midsummer Dionysian rite.

Except for the war in Vietnam, the fear of being drafted, and the three A's (angst, apocalypse, and alienation), college was a great experience. I loved it.

53

Classic Koch

The summer after freshman year I took no classes but held four part-time jobs, three of them concurrently. On a typical day I delivered the mail in Washington Heights at six in the morning. In the afternoon I took the subway to Grand Central and the Citizens Budget Commission, where I was supposed to improve the prose of the organization's press releases and reports but spent most of my time reading *Sons and Lovers* and Scott Fitzgerald. Saturday nights I donned a uniform and worked as a security guard at the rock and roll concerts in Forest Hills. That's how I got to see The Doors open for Simon and Garfunkel. The audience didn't much like The Doors but they did like the organ bars that kick off "Light My Fire," which you heard everywhere in 1967. My fourth job? I spent the last weeks of August back at Camp Harrow, where I was assigned to the youngest boys' bunk and charged with publishing the camp yearbook for distribution to the campers as they boarded the bus home on the last day.

Twice that summer, the summer of 1967, I went to an assembly room in Butler Library and listened to Kenneth Koch expound on two poems, "Blocks" by Frank O'Hara and "Our Youth" by John Ashbery. By then I considered myself a poet and a zealous convert to the poetics of the New York School. I had written a poem titled

"The Presidential Years," which won a university poetry prize and would appear in the *Paris Review*. And one day in the fall Associate Dean William Harlan, who taught the justly celebrated lecture course, "Conspiracies and Conspiracy Theories from Julius Caesar to JFK," summoned me to his office, congratulated me on making dean's list, and said that Columbia had awarded me a scholarship from a fund set up by Governor Nelson Rockefeller and former mayor Robert Wagner. My father and mother came to the auditorium to see me shake hands with Rocky.

Then came 1968.

That spring I hated the trendy course I took in radical social change but could bullshit my way through it, unlike the poor fellow who took exception to "ersatz proletarian posturing" and dropped the class. It was music humanities that gave me fits. I didn't make a sufficient effort to read music, didn't pay close enough attention in class; and then, because of campus protests and riots having nothing to do with music, classes were suspended. How to prepare for the final? It would be decisive in determining my grade. I went out and bought six or seven records: Bach's *Ein feste Burg ist unser Gott*; Mozart's *Jupiter Symphony*; Beethoven's Third, Fifth, and Seventh; Brahms's Fourth. I played these vinyl records multiple times on my stereo. My favorite was Beethoven's Seventh. I played it over and over. At the final the professor said he was going to play a portion of a piece we had not heard in class. The students had to do their best to identify the period of the piece and, if possible, its composer, and to explain our reasoning. There was a hush as we waited for the record to play. The needle hit the vinyl and the first notes of the slow movement of Beethoven's Seventh came out. A few days later, the professor phoned me to say, with some wonderment, that I had aced the exam. He invited me to his apartment for tea. He played the *Symphonie fantastique* and explained that

Berlioz had written it in an opium haze. "Was Berlioz the Baude-laire of music?" I asked. "Very good," he answered.

In 1968 I saw *Belle de Jour* in a midtown cinema and *The Cocktail Party* on Broadway, *The Importance of Being Earnest* in London, and *As You Like It* at Stratford-upon-Avon. I spent the summer in Oxford and visited Paris for the first time. In Florence I roomed with a fellow on the *Harvard Crimson* who read about the riots at the Democratic convention in Chicago and wished he'd been there.

On a February day in 1968, Columbia canceled all classes and proposed that we devote the day to a moratorium: classes would be suspended and, in their stead, there would be teach-ins and lectures about the war in Vietnam. I forget who the big name lecturers were but remember the poetry reading at Barnard that evening: Ted Berrigan read some of his sonnets, David Shapiro read Whitman's "Reconciliation" and a few poems of his own, Allen Ginsberg chanted and read, and Kenneth Koch dazzled the crowd with his sublimely funny, relentlessly affirmative poem "The Pleasures of Peace."

In 1968 I became a full-fledged disciple of "Vitamin K," one of Ashbery's nicknames for the most inspiring poetry instructor I have ever had or observed. I've seen Kenneth teach college students, little kids, and aged residents of nursing homes, and whatever the audience, he managed to get them excited about poetry, excited enough to write poems. If you were a writer at Columbia it didn't matter whether the course was nominally on seventeenth-century poetry or the comic in modern literature. You were taking a course in the mind of Kenneth Koch.

"You're a unique combination of naïveté and ambition," Kenneth told me at a party before introducing me to someone else, a painter, as his "spiritual grandfather." I think that everyone was Kenneth's "spiritual grandfather" that evening.

"What's your favorite shape?"

"Circle. What's yours?"

"Star. Your favorite word?"

"Eden."

"Mine is snob," he said, adding that he believed he had "won" the exchange. I remembered it years later when my wife and I took Kenneth to the only Italian restaurant in Clinton, New York. The waiter scooped up the menus.

"I'll be right back with the garlic bread," he said and went to the kitchen.

"As if they had garlic bread in Italy," Kenneth said with disdain when the waiter was out of earshot. Well, he had a point.

As an undergraduate at Harvard, Koch (pronounced like the soft drink) had taken lecture notes in ottava rima and written the answers to at least one final exam entirely in blank verse. In his classes, he was a virtuoso and a show-off, capable of making up a poem on the spot. To illustrate a point, Koch liked resorting to a quotation, often from a French poet. Mallarmé to Degas: Poems are made with words, not ideas. Paul Valéry: A poem is a communication from one who is not the poet to one who is not the reader. T. S. Eliot: It is possible to enjoy poetry before you understand it. Boris Pasternak: "The landscape lurched to a halt." Kenneth hated the words "creative writing" and "workshop" and he disliked the workshop model; he was the teacher and we did a lot more listening than talking. He said a few times that there were only five or six major truths and one of them was that the organs of sex and the organs of excretion are located in the same place. He came up with the most wonderful assignments. Imitate William Carlos Williams, Gertrude Stein, Borges. Turn a poem by Wordsworth into one by Wallace Stevens. Adopt Machado de Assis's narrative strategy. Write two different stories, both ending with the exact same sentence. Without consulting the play, write a plausible first scene for *Hamlet*. Buy a comic book, tape blank paper in the dialogue balloons, and substitute your own sentences. Write a poem in collaboration with a classmate. Write a sestina, a prose poem, a poem based on today's newspaper. Write a poem, then cut it up, scrambling the lines. Attempt a "sound" translation of a canto in Dante's *Inferno*. Put together a collage. Translate a poem by Arthur Rimbaud. The rationale of these assignments was all-important: you didn't have to wait for inspiration to strike. You could make it happen.

Koch hated bad poetry— *poésie,* he called it—as if it were a moral offense. Bad poetry was artificial, fake; it was full of pieties and lofty sentiments, it observed conventions that were weary, stale, flat, and unprofitable. The "roadkill" poem, for instance— the poem in which, Koch said, "the poet kills a deer and feels like a rat, or maybe he killed a rat and feels like a deer." With his antics and sometimes wild gesticulations Kenneth called to mind television's Sergeant Bilko hatching a plot designed to promote anarchy as an aesthetic act. His humor survived any amount of adversity. When, in the last year of his life, he was undergoing radical treatment for leukemia at the Anderson Cancer Center in Houston, he introduced a visitor to his IV pole. "I'd like to introduce you to Duchamp's sister," he said.*

* The visitor was the late poet Paul Violi.

54

The Poem Team

Mitch and Les, two of the editors of *Columbia Review*, dreamed up the Columbia "poem team" consisting of the magazine's regulars who would tour women's colleges—Sarah Lawrence, Vassar, and Mount Holyoke—and read our poems and stories. Would the Columbia administration support the effort with funds to cover gas and sundries? Because I was the most conventional looking of the group, I was drafted to pitch the idea to Associate Dean Erwin Glikes, who liked my wide brown paisley tie in the Peter Max manner. When the phone rang, he apologized and pointed to the couch in the office. On the table in front were various issues of a magazine called *The Second Coming*. The magazine printed poems by John Ashbery and Kenneth Koch.

"This is a great magazine," I said.

The statement delighted Erwin Glikes, who, unbeknownst to me, was an editor of *The Second Coming*. He approved the request for funds, chuckling and wondering if we wanted blue-and-white windbreakers with names and numbers on the back, a wonderful idea that went nowhere.

It was, I believe, Mitch who wrote the poem team's manifesto, which began with the proclamation that "a poem is not as valuable as a sheep."

Everyone wanted Mitch's approval. Chicago-born, he played lightweight football and hosted a radio program on the "Monsters of the Midway," the Chicago Bears in their glory years. Mitch had a wry sense of humor and a way of cracking himself up when telling a story that made the laughter contagious. One time he and another fellow were sitting on the ledge facing Ferris Booth Hall, which was then the student activities center with a movie theater, a bowling alley, and the Lion's Den, a café where you could eat hamburgers, drink coffee, and listen to the Supremes sing "You Keep Me Hangin' On." The fellow took a poem out of his pocket and showed it to Mitch, who read it, handed it back, and said, "Not one of your major works." That line was used pretty regularly after that.

Mitch wrote a series of one-line poems that started with one titled "I Am the Toilet." The line: "Dance on, you pigs. I will never get used to it."*

For the mimeographed daily the guys on the *Columbia Review* published under the title "Janet Benderman," the editors needed copy and Mitch's one-line poems were perfect for the purpose. Unfortunately, in those days before photocopy machines became commonplace, the original was lost and the only remnants were "I Am the Toilet" and the title, but not the text, of a second poem: "Cardinal Spellman's Big Day." The editors got around the problem by running today's title with yesterday's line: "Dance on, you pigs, I will never get used to it."

---

* I suspect he got the line from Kafka.

55

Shakespeare's Birthday

On April 4, 1968, Martin Luther King was assassinated.

On April 23, Shakespeare's birthday, a student protest at the Sundial on College Walk led to a march on the proposed site of the gymnasium the university was planning to build in Morningside Park. In the eyes of the protesters, the gym was an example of the university's self-aggrandizement, exploitation of the local community, and insensitivity to the residents of Harlem. That night rebellious students occupied Hamilton Hall, and for the following week five buildings ordinarily used for classrooms and administrative offices were held by protesters. There were no classes. Ad hoc faculty committees debated what should be done. The campus was overrun with reporters. People wore armbands. Green signified that you favored amnesty for the protesters, including those who took over the offices of the deans and kept those deans captive for twenty-four hours; white, that you were a noncombatant, a faculty or staff member solicitous of the welfare of the occupants; blue meant you belonged to the "majority coalition" that deplored the demonstrators and defended the university from charges of racism and complicity with the Defense Department; a red armband was worn by true believers in revolution, violent if necessary. After the police busted heads and cleared out the buildings a week later, there were many black armbands signifying lament for Alma Mater.

I saw Kenneth Koch on campus. "Come on, David. Tell the truth." He pointed to Low Memorial Library, where the offices of the university's president and provost were located. "Aren't the guys in there mainly to get laid?"

Inside Low Library my friend David Shapiro, maybe the most talented poet on campus (and Koch's favorite), seated himself in the president's chair wearing dark glasses and smoking a cigar, and the photograph appeared in *Life* as the face of the uprising.

On the night of the big bust, Mitch and I supped on sandwiches and beer at the West End Bar. We decided to interpose our bodies between the building's entrance and the rushing cops and were sitting next to each other in front of Avery Hall when the student protesters were evicted. These weren't just any cops. These were members of the TPF, the Tactical Patrol Force, elite warriors. It was a tense moment. Koch stood among the faculty cordon right in front of us. Mitch recited the Twenty-third Psalm (and, incongruously, Thomas Wyatt's sonnet "They Flee from Me") as we waited for the officers to come at us swinging their sticks. Reading about the bust in the *New York Times*, I learned for the first time that the newspaper of record is reliable except on subjects about which the reader knows a good deal.

Kathy S., a Barnard junior who wrote the best prose of any of us in Koch's writing class, was a proud occupant of Mathematics Hall. I spent one night in Mathematics to be near Kathy and got cornered into emceeing a poetry reading in the building the next afternoon. A doctor read an ode to Mickey Mantle's five hundredth home run. But one day inside was enough for me. Kathy wrote a terrific piece about the occupation. I put in a brief appearance as a character named Ted who is smitten with the author.

Although nothing exasperates a woman as much as unwanted advances from an importunate suitor, Kathy was as sweet to me as a woman in that position can be. Having spent a year in France, she introduced me to Chez Brigitte on Greenwich Avenue in the Village, where the omelettes were really French, and the two of us discovered La Petite Marmite in the West Fifties, where we feasted on canard à l'orange and a very cold Chablis. She told me that in France the vegetables, and not only the tomatoes, are like fruits. We met in Paris that summer, and when she left for the south, I moved from my hotel room near the Seine and rented hers, less expensive, on rue Toullier (I think) around the corner from the rue Soufflot, the hilly street at the top of which rested the Panthéon.

Kathy's father was a brain surgeon. In early June I stayed in the spare bedroom of her parents' place in Philadelphia after she and I saw a Bergman film, *Hour of the Wolf.* We must have looked suspicious because a cop stopped us in the street and asked us what we were doing and I improvised that we were out buying milk for our baby. Back in the city I turned on the news. It was the night of the California primary. I saw that Bobby Kennedy won the primary and turned off the set maybe sixty seconds too soon. The next morning I found out about the assassination. He was still alive but Kathy's father said he was a goner by the time he got to the hospital, and so he was.

56

Recovery Room

They kept me in the recovery room overnight. Here's how Stacey describes that night:

In addition to removing David's bladder, the surgeon explained that he took out dozens of surrounding lymph nodes. The margins were clear. "It's out," he said, referring to the cancer. This happy news would be confirmed by the pathology report.

Hours went by uneventfully. My brother-in-law left. My sister would have stayed but it was past eight in the evening. "We're waiting for his room," the receptionist said when I asked about David's status. The room still wasn't ready when the staff changed shift. As far as I could tell he was still in the recovery room. Had something gone wrong? And why couldn't I be with him?

I was alone in the waiting area. Everyone else had gone home. The room was decorated like a cheap chain motel lobby and the garbage bags overflowed with empty fast food containers and coffee cups. Boxes containing scattered slices of cold pizza covered the counter near the coffee machine.

"You can wait for him in his room," the OR receptionist said when I next approached her. "At last," I thought. She gave me the room number, but her counterpart on the urological floor had no record of David. The nurses wanted me to go home. "There's nothing you can do here," they said. "We'll let you know when he's released to his room."

I took the elevator to the recovery suite, but it was crowded and I seemed to be in the way so I took a seat in the corridor. While watching the nurses tend to David, I did something I rarely do: I burst into tears. "Why is this happening? Why isn't he in his room yet?"

Ms. Brady, the "patient advocate," went to find out. She returned with a smile on her face, her arms wide, as if she were going to embrace me.

"He's staying here tonight," she said. "In recovery. Doctor's orders." She was ebullient. It didn't make sense. What was there to be happy about? "Now you absolutely must go home," she said. "You can't stay here all night."

Why not? And why is he still in the recovery room?

It was, I am convinced, by virtue of my hysteria and doggedness that I finally got an answer. Because of the scary "heart block" of last December, the cardiologist ordered that David be closely observed through the night. If all went well, he would be released to a room in the morning. The orders had been in his chart all along but nobody had told us.

"Do you work there?" the cab driver said as we headed downtown.

"No. My husband is a patient."

"My sister died there," he said. "Of stomach cancer." He proceeded to tell me about the guilt he still felt because he couldn't pay for the care she needed.

Everyone has a cancer story.

57

The Rebbe

On my third day after radical surgery I met the rebbe. "In what language do you prefer to speak," he wanted to know. He was fluent in Yiddish, Hebrew, English, and, I suspect, Russian and French.

"In Yiddish we do not have a word for this disease," he said.

"What do you call it?" I asked.

"We call it the disease we are forbidden to name."

I had a private room so Stacey could stay with me round the clock. She slept in a fold-out cot. After the surgeon's morning rounds, she left for our apartment downtown to shower and change. Having been poked and prodded by a parade of doctors, nurses, aides, I was usually asleep by the time she returned. On this day she shook me out of my morphine-induced fog. "There's a *minyan* on the other side of the floor," she told me. "Let's take an old-fashioned walk."

If I wanted to be released from the hospital, I had to be able to circumnavigate the floor at least ten times. "Don't fade into the sheets," the surgeon said.

I shuffled around the corridor attached to my IV pole, nodding in solidarity to other patients engaged in the same ballet, all wearing the same threadbare hospital gowns, unselfconscious about the open backs that revealed pale, flabby buttocks. We pass the nurse's station, where, depending upon who is working, I may get a "Good for you!" or even a little flirtatious banter with Nurse Engel, my favorite. Then comes the hot-blanket station, a glass-fronted cabinet stacked with coverlets. Hospitals are cold in every sense, and those warm blankets are a *mechayeh*, which is Yiddish for a bucket of ice water on a hike in the scorching Negev desert.

It takes a while to complete a circuit of the floor, with each step seeming to require a separate act of will. Just after the third right-angle turn, I passed the hospital room of Rabbi Aharon Eliezer Ceitlin, who (I learned) had been flown in from Israel with all his family thanks to donations from Hasidic communities around the world. A group of bearded Hasidim in their white beards, black suits, black hats, and prayer fringes stood around speaking in low tones. Themselves rabbis of note, they had come from various cities to show their respect, to pray with the famous rebbe, and to hear what he would have to say.

Like me, Rabbi Ceitlin was hooked up to an IV pole. Though gaunt, he was a large man. He wore wire-rim glasses that did nothing to diminish the bright intensity of his dark-brown eyes. He bade me join the group in prayers. Someone found me a seat. Stacey held back, knowing the Orthodox custom of separating men from women, but they waved her in. She introduced herself with her Hebrew name, Shoshana. The day happened to be the *yahrzeit* of the greatly revered Menachem Mendel Schneerson (1902–1994), the last rebbe of the Lubavitcher Hasidic dynasty, so the rabbis were *davening* with particular fervor. In 1976, Rabbi Schneerson had hand-picked the young Rabbi Ceitlin to be an emissary to Israel. It was an inspired choice. Over the years Rabbi Ceitlin worked tirelessly to promote Jewish education. He established a network of Chabad kindergartens, thirty-four in all, serving 1,500 children in the ancient city of Safed.

Someone lent me a yarmulke and a *tallis*. We chanted *mincha*. Then Rabbi Ceitlin delivered a commentary. He told of a wealthy man who came to the rabbi for advice. The man, a congregant who gave generous sums for *tzedakah*, wanted to know whether he was "on the right level" in his relationship with God. *On the right level!* The rabbi couldn't help laughing at the phrase, and I joined in the laughter, loudly. What did the rabbi tell the man? He told the man that he should wake up tomorrow, go to work, do your duty, observe the commandments, spend time with your family.

"That was the first time you've laughed in I don't know how long," Stacey said later.

"He got it," the rebbe announced to the room when I laughed with him, and I still think the anecdote is hilarious though it mystifies every friend with whom I've shared it.

Later, when we were alone, Rabbi Ceitlin wanted to know how I made a living. I told him I was the author of books. "And you can make a living doing that?" He complimented me on my Hebrew, rusty as it is, and patiently corrected each error of pronunciation I made as I read a prayer. He shook my hand. In that hospital room I felt I was in sacred space.

The next day the rabbi's son visited me in my room. "My father would like you to pray with him," he said. "And if it isn't something you want to do for yourself, it would still be a *mitzvah* for you to let him pray with you." I went. I didn't have *tefillin* so Rabbi Ceitlin let me wear his. I asked about his condition and he asked about mine.

"The waiting is difficult," he said. "Even Moses complained about having to wait. 'A little longer and they will stone me,' Moses said."

The rebbe told me about the legendary Reb Levik, the spiritual leader of a great Hasidic community in an unpronounceable Ukrainian city. A stranger entered Reb Levik's shul and when he looked to his right, he saw everyone rise. Then he looked to his left, and the same thing happened. The stranger was astonished. Then he saw Reb Levik himself—not an assistant or a functionary, mind you, but the great Reb Levik himself—stride down the aisle to hand him a *siddur*. The congregation had stood in honor of the beloved rabbi. But some of that honor was meant for the stranger, the *"Yiddishe neshama,"* Rabbi Ceitlin said, knowing that "Jewish soul" could not convey the import of that Yiddish phrase.

This was in June, the third of Tammuz in the Hebrew calendar. On October 15, Rabbi Aharon Eliezer Ceitlin passed away.

58

Life Begins at Forty

When the doctors discharged me after seven nights in the hospital, I couldn't have been happier. I had worked out with a physical therapist, an occupational therapist, done the exercises, proved that I could manage in the bathroom by myself. But I looked shaky, pale. A man in a uniform hailed me a cab.

A week has gone by. It is one in the afternoon. A burst of intense pain interrupts my reverie and I lie in bed for twenty minutes, get up, steady myself, and go to the computer to write my five hundred words of the day.

Each year of your life is a microcosm of the whole. That is my assumption.

If you could return to any year in your life, which would you choose?

I'd probably pick 1988, the year I turned forty, the year when life, real life, is supposed to begin.

Here are a dozen or so things I remember from 1988:

In the Ear Inn in 1988, I went into the unisex bathroom and read the graffiti. A graffito from 1980 had been erased: "Support your local philosopher. Buy a jockstrap."

In Miami, on a visit to my mother, I got to spend a little time with Isaac Bashevis Singer. He made great claims for the sexual organs. "An eye will not stop seeing if it doesn't like what it sees, but the penis will stop functioning if he doesn't like what he sees. I would say that the sexual organs express the human soul more than any other limb of the body. They are not diplomats. They tell the truth ruthlessly."

Sitting at my mother's desk, writing a few lines, signing a few checks. I opened the drawer and there were forty-year-old paper clips. There was pleasure in using a pencil that was new in 1948.

I discovered a story I had written in college. It began with a sweeping authoritative observation: "People duplicate the same living room in all the apartments of their lives." Nineteen years and twelve apartments later, it was still true.

About progress my mother said, "Progress is sometimes too much already."

In February 1988, I made a splash and a boatload of permanent academic enemies when *Newsweek* ran my article on deconstructionist guru Paul de Man's posthumous disgrace because of his wartime journalism in favor of the Nazis in his native Belgium. One of the Yale professor's most ardent disciples had a nervous breakdown on hearing the news. Her uncle, a publishing executive, was among the first to make an offer for the book Glen suggested I write—*Signs of the Times*, though I didn't have that title when I wrote up the proposal in 1988.

In March, Glen and I flew to Phoenix, I to cover spring training for *Newsweek*, he to sign up Roger Craig for a book about the split-fingered fastball. We got to watch games and dine with Roger Angell, who had a new book that season. I asked Roger if he thought anyone would ever break Roger Maris's record of sixty-one home runs. He pointed to a player in an Oakland A's uniform and said, "If anyone can do it, it's Mark McGwire with that sweet, short swing." McGwire did it ten years later when he played for the

St. Louis Cardinals in 1998. He hit seventy home runs that year, though the prestige of that mark has suffered from the fact that McGwire played "during the steroid era," in his words, and used performance-enhancing drugs.

A. Bartlett Giamatti, president of the National League, formerly president of Yale, gave a press conference and all the beat reporters in their straw hats asked about the possibility of a female umpire in the majors. The barrel-chested Giamatti wore a loud red shirt with a massive gold chain around his neck. I raised my hand and asked for his thoughts about the Paul de Man scandal, and he spoke animatedly for five minutes, during which time all the beat reporters left. "Now look what you've done," Giamatti said. "Who are you anyway?" It was an enjoyable conversation. When I told Roger Angell about it, he said Bart will probably become commissioner, and a damn good one, too, if he doesn't keel over and die of a heart attack with all that weight he's carrying. Giamatti did become commissioner and had exactly the fate Angell predicted.

In April, I had lunch with Edward Said at the Columbia Faculty Club. As a widely admired literary theorist, he had a complete set of de Man's wartime articles, which the deconstructionist faithful were trying to keep from people like me. Edward had his assistant photocopy the whole thing, and I had it by the end of the day. He disliked de Man from the time they'd had a showdown at a summer conference devoted to "criticism and theory." Edward had spoken in favor of the world's objective existence while de Man argued in favor of "bracketing" all that. An intellectual disagreement, but Edward's ire suggested that it was the academic equivalent of a knockdown brawl.

In October we lunched again and Edward said that in the presidential contest he favored Jesse Jackson. "Well, that's not going to happen." I smiled. "And between Dukakis and Bush?" Edward shrugged his shoulders. "*Ça m'est égal,*" he said, signaling his indifference in French, perhaps to salute the time, seventeen years earlier, when he and I squared off at the pinball machine at Le Rond-Point, our go-to café, gone now, near the corner of Montparnasse and Raspail in Paris. Said was a very competitive pinball player.

In November, *The Best American Poetry 1988*—the first in the series—was published, and to everyone's surprise, including mine, three printings sold out before pub date.

In December, looking for cover art, I asked Larry Rivers how he differs from Andy Warhol. Larry showed me one of his "smudge" paintings inspired by a Dutch Masters cigar box. Then he showed me a box of Dutch Masters. "What Warhol does is more like what the cigar manufacturer did." We used a Rivers painting of Fred Astaire on the cover of the 1989 *Best American Poetry*.

We were on the way to Seton Hall in New Jersey where I was to mediate a conversation with Larry and John Ashbery. In the car John said he was reading the paperback of Vanna White's memoir on the toilet. There was a quiet moment. Then he looked out the window and said: "Look at the lovely older homes here."

59

Search for Meaning

Today I translated a poem from the German that doesn't exist:
Heinrich Heine's "Search for Meaning." A footnote in Freud's
Civilization and Its Discontents had led me to it.

I kept looking for the meaning of life
But I couldn't find it anywhere
I looked in books
Tolstoy, Dostoyevsky, Nietzsche, Goethe, Dante.
Surely, they must have the answer
But they didn't and I went to bed and had dreams in which
I searched for the meaning of life.
I turned to philosophers,
But do they teach you how to live?
I went to Japan, to India, hoping I would find the answer
In a pond or in a cave but when I threw a rock
Or shouted my name the echoes were overwhelming
And the ripples in the pond perplexed me.
In Philosophy 101, the professor said "the meaning of life"
Is a nonsense phrase and the same goes for "Eden" and "paradise"
By logic he proved that life was meaningless
But I didn't believe it I decided to get drunk
I went to the *cabaret vert* that night
The legs of the tango dancer were magnificent

But they weren't the meaning of life
Her eyes were real, though she used liner and shadow
Her lips were real though she used lipstick
She wore a double strand of pearls with earrings to match
And as I sipped my drink I knew
The search for the meaning of life would have to wait.

60

The Old Religion

Three weeks have gone by since the surgery. I can barely sum-mon up the strength to walk around the block or climb a flight of stairs. For my peripheral neuropathy, I can offer you a choice of similes: it's as if your feet were encased in cement or, on better days, as if your toes were webbed together. It is July, and hot, but when I walk into an air-conditioned store I have to walk right out—it makes me shiver. I have lost thirty pounds. Tomorrow they are going to remove the staples and it is going to hurt like hell. But I insist on my hour or two at the computer. And I don't want to use these words, this space, to bitch about the indignities and trials of the day.

"How can I help?" "You can ask questions or give answers." Long pause. I have another cup of orange pekoe tea. For almost a year now I have not been able to drink coffee. It occurs to me to wonder about the English national character, about which Orwell writes in "England Your England." In my own time over there the English drank tea, not coffee, and if that has changed, if it is now difficult to find an honest-to-goodness pot of tea, brewed from the leaves, not tea bags ("instant tea"), it makes me wonder whether the change reflects a change in the very character of that great island people. What I liked about England was that it was different from the US. Now it's more of the same.

Finally you get a word in edgewise: "Do you remember the first time it was explained to you that you are Jewish and therefore different from other people?"

Yes, we were standing on the corner of Arden Street and Sherman Avenue and I asked my father: Why do we wear hats in the street? "Because we are Jews and this is how we show respect for God."

Religion preceded almost everything else in my consciousness of the external manmade world—of society, the system, the status quo, things as they are.

Everyone in the school I went to was the son or daughter of refugees from Hitler's Europe—what we now call "Holocaust survivors." Some had numbers tattooed on their arms. In the street there were plenty of fistfights between the Catholic kids and the Christkillers. We were also sheenies and yids, and sometimes when Mr. Moran and his eldest son, Edward, who lived down the hall from us, came back stinking from the tavern on a Friday night, they hurled loud threatening drunken curses at the Jews. You could hear them a block away.

My father's siblings and their families were true to their high Orthodox upbringing. My father was more lenient than his siblings. My mother's side of the family was more casual in the observance. She, her brother Bert, and cousins Rita and Bina remained Viennese all their lives, like children who didn't need something to be funny in order to laugh.

On walks in Fort Tryon Park my father explained the cosmos, the planets, and the continents. I learned about Hitler at an early age. On the black clock radio in the kitchen came a chorus singing pack up your troubles in your old kit bag and smile smile smile. At the kitchen table with the red-and-white-checkered tablecloth my mother served pancakes Hungarian style, very thin and delicious with raspberry jam. She told us about our new cousin we were going to meet. He and his mother had been rescued from Yugoslavia, where the boy's father had been killed. "By the Reds," the boy said tersely. He played guitar for us and sang in Serbian.

Before I went to Cambridge, my father and I had one of our late-night heart-to-hearts in the living room. When I told him about the Cambridge tripos, he sat back in his green reclining armchair, closed his eyes, and savored the thought of my spending leisurely hours looking at Tintorettos and Titians, taking part in a Shakespeare play, walking in the tutors' gardens of Clare and Pembroke, living the life of a young gentleman—something he, a refugee businessman, had never had the chance to do. My father winked at me once, when I punned on the French word for *arm*, and I suspect there were days when he contented himself with enjoying my life from afar. Some of my happiest times on earth were when I felt I had not his approval so much as his enjoyment of my escapades and my education as he imagined these things to be.

61

The Problem of Evil

As Dostoyevsky wrote, everyone lies about himself, even Rousseau in his *Confessions*, who, out of sheer vanity, confessed to crimes he did not commit.

By my reckoning, the plot summary of a well-loved movie can qualify as an autobiography and so can a theological meditation, a made-up story, a choice quotation, the summary of an unwritten book or movie never made, a close reading of a passage of prose, a rambling journal entry, a statement that sparks a chain of insights.

For example, today I was reading *Paradise Lost* when I had a thought that I wrote on the last page of the book:

The real question is not whether you believe in god as such but whether you believe there is such a thing as evil—evil as a choice, a matter of character and will, and not a mere reflection of environment.

62

Dean Martin's Hat

At the Las Vegas hospital, night shift were taking bets on the exact moment certain terminally ill cancer patients would kick the bucket. Good sporting proposition, but the lottery was fixed. Head nurse, in cahoots with an underling, pulls plug on life-support system at just the right moment, and the intensive care ward explodes like the victorious home crowd at the seventh game of the World Series.

Baudelaire: "Life is a hospital where the patients keep changing beds."

The wards have individual booths where the patients can watch nonstop cable television news while they drink the vile concoction that will illuminate their internal organs when their bodies slide into the X-ray cylinder for their CAT scans. On arriving I am complimented on my fedora: a two-toned black-and-brown Stetson from (I would guess) the early 1960s. I agree with the French critic who said that the most interesting thing about *Some Came Running* is Dean Martin's hat, which he wears even in bed, even in a hospital bed. But he demands his release though the doctor says his condition is very serious indeed. Diabetes, possibly terminal. And you have to give up drinking. That'll be the day. And then gunshots that were meant for Frank Sinatra kill Shirley MacLaine.

It's an incoherent movie, and the song that Sammy Cahn and Jimmy Van Heusen wrote for it gets sung by a bland roadhouse trio, not FS (though he did record it memorably). But Dean Martin's hat is the best joke in the movie, and not just because it's the only one.

63

740 Francs

We desperately needed a new urologist. Stacey knew that Patti Hansen and her husband, Keith Richards, kept a duplex apartment (with four bedrooms and three private terraces) on high floors of our building in New York City. Having learned that Patti is a spokesperson for bladder cancer patients, Stacey got in touch with her, and Patti returned the call. She recommended the doctor who treated her. When she referred to him affectionately by his nickname, I knew this was the way to go. That conversation with Patti Hansen was a lifesaver. Stacey treasures the two-page handwritten letter she received from Keith in response to her telling him that she admired his memoir.

Stacey and I are often asked how we met. Sometimes I say that we served on a jury together and persuaded the rest of the jurors to see the case our way. Sometimes she says she had a local TV talk show and interviewed me for it. One time she told that story and the listener claimed to have watched the program.

We never tell people about the walks we took in the snow and the songs we sang together when we donned cross-country skis and spent the early morning crossing a field in the snow. We have our secrets. We don't mention the visit we made to the jewelry store. We do not speak about the night when we went to a small party, absented ourselves, ostensibly to use an ATM but in reality to cab it to my place in the Village, celebrate life, and return to the party with no one the wiser. I forget what excuse we used. Then there was the day of raincoats and umbrellas and the French bistro that lasted only a year on MacDougal Street just south of Bleecker. There were hotels in three states. At least four in New York City. One time we stayed at the Wales and were given room 619, a happy omen. But we don't speak about that.

We don't talk about it but we still revel in the honeymoon in Paris when she had her first glass of red wine after nine years of abstinence and we went with a camera and photographed every Paris residence Ashbery lived in—her idea. On John's recommendation we stayed at La Louisiane on the rue de Seine. From our second-floor oval *chambre* we could see the intersection of three streets. That first night, after sleeping, we walked over to the Deux Magots and drank tea outside under the heated lights. "Come on," I said. "Let's walk to the cathedral." We crossed the street and on the corner of Saint-Germain-des-Prés we looked down and there were 740 French francs on the pavement. That week we went to Le Dôme and visited with Lelia Tchistoganow, who had been the director of Columbia's Parisian outpost, Reid Hall, when my buddies and I lived there. And we were photographed in the garden and then we took a walk and found the little street where Apollinaire wrote his poem "Lundi rue Christine." There was a restaurant on the right side as you walked down the curved street toward the Seine. We walked in, ate foie gras, drank a fine Sauterne, and signed the guest book with a flourish like lovers who didn't mind who knew it.

64

Shalom Aleichem Rides to the Rescue

The question was: How are you going to get out of the draft?

In my senior year of college I had a low draft number in the lottery and was nervous about having to go to Vietnam. Morris Simon, father of Rochelle, the curly-haired brunette on whom I had a crush, was considered the wise man of the synagogue, and it was to him that my father suggested I go to for advice. Mr. Simon was the head of the temple's Chevra Kadisha, which undertook the community's funeral arrangements and cemetery maintenance. After I had my say, he made this cheerful little speech.

"There's really nothing to worry about," he said. "You have to go to the army. Well, one of two things will happen. Either you'll be sent to Vietnam or you won't. If you're not, what's there to worry about? But let's say they send you to Vietnam. One of two things will happen. You'll get a cushy desk job in Saigon or you'll go to the front. If you get the desk job, there's nothing to worry about. But even suppose they volunteer you into the 173rd Airborne Brigade and God forbid they send you to the Mekong Delta as part of Operation Marauder and there are two short artillery rounds and you get wounded and the helicopter comes for you, one of two things will happen. Either you'll recover or you won't. If you recover, what's there to worry about? But even suppose you don't recover, one of two things will happen. You'll be buried in hallowed ground like a good Jewish boy or you won't. If you're buried in hallowed ground, what's there to worry about? But even suppose you're not buried in hallowed ground. Well," Mr. Simon paused, "well, then, my dear fellow, you're in one hell of a fix."

65

The Arrival of the Messiah

It was the week before Passover, Shabbat Hagadol in the Hebrew calendar, and my father said a few words on the subject of the week's *haftorah*, which is taken from the third chapter of Malachi. The arrival of the Messiah is announced and the blessed are rewarded for their faith and their studious indifference to material gains. On them shall shine the glory of the Lord. True wealth goes not to those who seek but to those who believe. In the dark the courtesan has charms that dwarf those of the queen. But in the light of day there is no comparison.

My father opened his annotated Tanakh and read from the Rambam's commentary. "The queen gleams like an emerald set in gold. And in the light of day when the Messiah comes it will become clear who has royal blood, the princess empurpled in furs with her face painted garishly or the devout woman who called no attention to herself but was humble in the face of the Lord. The true queen in this parable is the Sabbath, the sweet rest at the end of the week, which is all the reward the virtuous man aspires to have—to take a nap in the afternoon and not to be interrupted."

"Amen," my mother said.

My father closed the book and softened his tone. "Do you remember the passage in Jeremiah in which the prophet wonders why the pious suffer while the wicked flourish?"

"Chapter twelve, verse one," my aunt Esther said.

"David and I have translated these lines using modern literary principles."

All eyes were on me.

"David, will you recite the passage for us?"

Now I understood why my father asked me to have a copy on hand of our collaborative work in progress. Taking the folded-up paper out of my inside breast pocket, I explained that Gerard Manley Hopkins has a great sonnet on the same theme from Jeremiah and so we lifted his first line for this effort.

> Thou art indeed just O Lord if I contend with thee,
> as wrestling I did once and blessed was
> though wounded in the hollow of my thigh.
> The Lord is just and yet I suffer.
> The rich traduce and yet they prosper,
> while I, who keep the faith of the fathers,
> must pray lest I stray from the righteous path.
> Stiffen my neck, Sir. Make my skin tougher.

Everyone murmured their approval. I gave my copy to my aunt Esther, who was so taken with the effort that she mailed me, a few weeks later, a much-thumbed copy of Erich Auerbach's *Mimesis,* along with a nice note saying that the importance of that book's first chapter would not be lost on one who had studied Jeremiah and Gerard Manley Hopkins as I had done. She was right about the greatness of the opening essay in Auerbach's book. But then I never knew Esther Lehman to be wrong on such matters.

66

Sabbath Services

The next morning I went to temple with my father. My favorite moment in the services came when the Torah was returned to the ark after the week's portion had been sung. The prayer is based on a line in Proverbs: "She is a tree of life to those who take hold of her; those who hold her fast will be blessed." Beautiful, too, the song in praise of the Lord chanted solemnly by the mourners on the anniversary of the loved one's death. *Yisgadal v'yiskadash sh'mei rabbaw.* Magnified and sanctified be the name of the Creator.

Next came the sermon. Our rabbi, Rabbi Kauffmann, the son of a Talmudic scholar famous in the old country, wore a black ceremonial skullcap of the finest silk brocade and was gloriously bearded in an age when mainly eccentrics or beatniks wore beards. He was a large man, somewhat remote in the German manner, who glowered with high dignity on all ceremonial occasions and had a thunderous voice. In his strict view all children born in America remained children even after they had gone off to college or the army. The rabbi's weekly sermons held me spellbound, though invariably just as he reached the climax, the moment for the moral or the epiphany, he would leave us hanging. He nearly always ended too abruptly—one or two sentences short of a satisfactory resolution. Then he would say, *"Heute und für alle Zeit. Amen"*—"Today and at all times. Amen"—even if that phrase had no logical or grammatical connection to the words that preceded it.

Usually he spoke in German, but on this day Rabbi Kauffmann made a speech in English about a man who was arrested for no reason. He had done nothing wrong. Yet he stood before the gates of justice and was unable to enter. Was he guilty before the law, and was this the plight of modern man, presumed guilty until proved innocent, and where would you get the proof of innocence if you didn't know the terms of the indictment? This wasn't the way of the Lord. This was the way of the secret police. Yet the sages tell us that the man thus accused was a pious and humble man, an ordinary god-fearing man, one of us. *Today and at all times. Amen.*

After services, I stood outside shaking hands with friends. Jeffrey Brenner was talking animatedly about Andy Bathgate of the New York Rangers, who had scored a goal on a penalty shot two nights previous at Madison Square Garden. Jeff had married Janice Klein, who was pregnant now with the couple's first child. Well, that was one way to beat the draft. Fathers were exempt. "How's married life?" "Couldn't be better," he said. Jeff, a compulsive joke-teller, had recently been hired to write "irony-of-fate-type" stories for Walter Cronkite at CBS News. I congratulated him on the job and he rolled his eyes. "You know, blind girl wins spelling bee. Republican flack marries Democratic congressman. Dachau survivor wins German lottery. You like that one? Okay. Dachau survivor wins German lottery. So he cleans up his act, goes on a diet, loses fifty pounds, gets a haircut, shaves, buys new threads. And then a car hits him when he crosses the street, and he lies there and says, God, why did you do this to me? And God says, Harry—for the man's name is Harry—to tell you the truth I didn't recognize you. And the tag line is, 'And that's the way it is.' Haw." Out of the corner of my eye, I can see Mrs. Kauffmann, the rabbi's wife, and I go over to pay my respects and to ask after her daughter Hannah, now at Stanford studying art history. Now *there* was a girl to marry and start a family with, I thought, before reminding myself that this couldn't and wouldn't happen. Her parents had ruled me out from the day I stopped observing the Sabbath and Jewish dietary laws.

Had I lived at home through college, kept kosher and observed the Sabbath with my father as in the old days—had I wooed Hannah and won her, gone to temple and laughed at jokers like Jeff—had I steered clear of drugs, Rimbaud, and avant-garde art, yes, this was one of the lives I could have lived but didn't. One of the one hundred autobiographies.

67

A Complicated Guy

I feel sick. On Facebook today somebody dismissed the Holocaust as "white-on-white crime" and therefore not worth getting all hung up over.

It has been three weeks since I made an entry. If I am unlucky I need to get up six times in the night and I cannot find the floor and I must run to the bathroom. If I am lucky I return to sleep and stay asleep past noon, dreaming that Hillary Clinton has sounded me out for advice on contemporary poetry or that I am a guest at a resort in Pearl Harbor and cannot find a working toilet.

I've lost another ten pounds. Stacey and other truth tellers say I look frail and sickly. My pharmacist friend George, an uninhibited fellow, goes so far as to say I look like a "dead man walking." Lately, whenever we're driving and the car hits a bump, a searing pain shoots up my flank. "Why don't they repair these roads!"

Then one night I can't sleep and in the morning, watching the news, I begin to shiver and shake.

"Why am I shaking?" I ask Stacey.

Let her tell it.

I was supposed to go to the gym for an early class and afterward meet Stefanie for lunch but I woke up late and wasn't feeling social so I canceled. I wonder what would have happened had I stuck to my original plan and been out of the house that morning.

 David came upstairs as usual but complained that he hadn't slept so instead of sitting in his chair to watch the news on TV, he lay down on the sofa. Within moments, his entire body was shaking violently. He was burning up. I called Stefanie and asked her to come over with a thermometer though I already knew that his fever had spiked. I phoned Memorial Sloan Kettering, and they told me to get to a hospital. Stefanie and I took him to the emergency room in Ithaca. She spent the whole of that day at our side.

The head nurse took one look and rushed the patient to an examination room. "You're scaring me," she said.

After a while the doctor came in to explain that one of David's kidneys was enlarged and that it was best for him to go to Upstate Medical in Syracuse. "You're a complicated guy," the doctor said, referring to David's rearranged insides. He called for an ambulance to take David and me to Syracuse. Now that we had a plan, I urged Stefanie to go home. We had arrived at the hospital in the early afternoon and now it was past nine o'clock and dark outside. She kissed David's forehead. "I love you," she said, and typing this just now moves me to tears. She was and is beyond wonderful.

Hours later the ambulance arrived. The ambulance driver had served in the marines and was, in his words, a Hemingway aficionado.

Always have a "go bag" ready with everything you need in case of an emergency. Not yet having learned that lesson, I arrived at the emergency room wearing only a sundress and flip-flops. At the last minute I grabbed my telephone charger.

 At first, the doctors in Syracuse refused to call David's surgeon in New York City in order to coordinate treatment.

 "Do it now," I said. "I've phoned them and they're expecting your call."

 I got my way. Dr. M. phoned Dr. B. in NYC and the latter approved the former's plan, which was to treat David with heavy-duty antibiotics in the expectation that the swelling in his kidney would go down on its own and he wouldn't need an invasive procedure to drain it.

With the pen and paper they provided, he busied himself writing similes: "The next three days went by at the speed of a tortoise saving his energy for the final kick."

If my accounting here makes it seem like I was stalwart and in control, you've been misled. I was a mess. David was asleep for most of the time and I couldn't stop crying. I alternated between calling my sister and calling David's friend Glen. Both were able to calm me down in their way. Glen is calm and forceful, matter-of-fact and sensible. Amy is reassuring. At one point, she talked me through a breathing exercise and gave me sound advice: "Go to the nurses' station, tell them you're having a panic attack, and ask to see the hospital social worker." This was day three. I hadn't showered or slept for more than a fitful couple of hours. I was still in my sundress and flip-flops though I could stay warm with a hospital blanket.

The social worker led me to a small private room where I broke down completely. Dr. M. joined us and I confessed that I thought that David would die. "Here? Now?" Dr. M. sounded incredulous. "Don't you think he'd be in intensive care if we thought that was a possibility?" I had to admit he made sense. The social worker arranged for me to have a shower and a change of clothes. My doctor called in a prescription for anti-anxiety medication and for the first time in days I was able to sleep.

Two days later, David was released. Glen drove up from NYC to take us home and stayed the night. He was gone before I woke up the next morning, and later that day I noticed that before leaving he had pruned some of our bushes. I love Glen.

Stefanie, so vital in this narrative, is the mother of my son. So it was my wife and my ex-wife who saw me to the hospital, and it was Glen, my literary agent and close friend, who came through in the clutch.

Now you know why I feel blessed.

68

The Patient Next to You

In the army it is name, rank, and serial number. In the hospital it is name and birthday. Otherwise there are very striking similarities between these two hierarchical structures in which you, whoever you are, forfeit your identity and become either a soldier or a patient. Like an infantryman, the patient is fighting boredom most of the time, waiting and figuring out ways to pass the hours until the wait is over.

Just as you've dozed off, a nurse turns on all of the lights in your room and an orderly wheels in another patient; what had been a private room is now shared with the newcomer and several members of his frantic family. The poor guy was mauled by a cow. This is how you know that you're not in New York City but in a hospital that serves rural New York. "She tossed him around like he was a rag doll," his wife tells the doctor. He is strapped to a gurney, immobile, with a broken neck, back, and several broken ribs. He is crying and moaning. The coming and going is constant. The doctor explains that the cowherd will need surgery but that it's risky. More crying.

In your fevered state you believe that he dies behind the curtain and his wife and daughter sob and they wheel his bed out of the room with a sheet on top and all you can think about is the noise they are making and you are desperate to return to sleep.

After walking as instructed from your room to the nurses' station and back, you feel that you need to sleep for three hours, and when you wake, there is a different stranger in the second bed in the room, and you go back to sleep and in your dream he, too, dies, and when you wake and you see him alive you sound cheerful and he asks you why and you decide not to explain what happened to the predecessor in his bed.

Then something goes haywire with your gastrointestinal system.

Dr. Weingarten comes in and explains what went wrong with the last test and why they'll have to redo it. "You may feel some discomfort," he says. "Nothing you can't handle." He asks you to list your symptoms but interrupts after the first three. "I have a right to be arrogant," he says, because infectious diseases are his specialty. A nurse takes the paperwork to the laboratory and the results are inconclusive and you walk around the ward with your IV pole and your gown that opens from the back, and a pretty Italian nurse flirts with you as you circumnavigate the ward and when you get back to your room there is Dr. Weingarten again.

"Look," he says. "I'm nothing if not honest. The whole thing got screwed up. When I put the order in I specified 'clenicollect.' They had no record of it at Lab Corp."

"But I thought you said my test is negative."

"Your test is negative but negative for only one of the two toxins."

"I see," I said, though I didn't.

"What can I say? I take ownership of it."

I say nothing.

"Life isn't perfect. I need you to take the test again."

That means a third time. He recognizes that it is not a fun test and he is sorry. He leaves you with the paperwork and after he leaves, you take a quick look at it. It has someone else's name, not yours, and the test requested is for AIDS.

There are two popular American ways you can react to routine screwups and maintain your newly achieved equanimity. You can quote (a) Hyman Roth, "I said to myself this is the business we have chosen. I didn't ask who gave the order, because it had nothing to do with business," or (b) the wisdom of the elders: "So things go, at three in the morning, in some small dive."

69

Cambridge

If I close my eyes and concentrate, I can still do it, can still picture myself in my rooms in Clare College's Memorial Court on an early autumn day. There's a framed reproduction of a Matisse still life with oysters on the wall. On the record player I may be playing Beethoven's Ninth, Dvořák's *New World Symphony*, Rimsky-Korsakov's *Scheherazade*, Bartók's *Concerto for Orchestra*, Mozart's clarinet quintet, Stravinsky's *Firebird* and *The Rite of Spring*. My turquoise Smith-Corona is on my desk with a sheet of paper in it. There's an armchair and beside it a small table with an ashtray and the books I am reading this week, *Death in Venice*, *The Immoralist*, *The Birth of Tragedy*, *Emma*, Virginia Woolf, Rilke's poems, Ashbery's *Double Dream of Spring*, and the prematurely titled *Complete Poems* of Elizabeth Bishop.

If Oxford is towers and spires, Cambridge is birds and bells. If you love birdsong, you will love Cambridge in the early morning hours. A parliament of birds convenes outside your window and you hear their excitement at the light flooding the courtyard. They sing you awake as if you were in the Middle Ages and they were in Nottingham or Sherwood Forest having adventures and whispering in the ear of their favorite hero, a boy who whistles his way to safety. The bells mark the hours with melodies or the trace of melodies, like Schubert's *Military March* or the opening of the fourth movement of Mozart's *Jupiter Symphony*, which I am always hearing if I listen for it.

Your song in my ears, ye birds, I walk across the Clare College bridge, not only the oldest but the finest of all the bridges along "the Backs" of the river Cam, with the stone balls on top and the arches below, and then I enter the main courtyard, walk across to the porter's lodge, pick up my mail, read it in the seventeenth century, then turn around, retracing my steps, only this time I turn sharply right after crossing the bridge into the twentieth century, and now I am strolling in the most magnificent garden in this town of glorious gardens and Gothic gates. I marvel at how much art goes into the arrangements of flowers and bushes and trees, and yet how skillfully the artifice is concealed. Unlike a French homage to symmetry and Cartesian principle, this garden is nature glorified, not subjugated. It is as nature itself would be if she could afford a royal retinue of retainers. Here are gardens within gardens enclosed by clipped yew hedges leading to yet other gardens on paths lined with blue spruces. The deep green of the lawn with twin-sided herbaceous border; the apple trees with their ripening fruit, green on the road to red, dropping off the branches; the burst of red and orange and yellow flowers along the banks of the Cam; the sunken pond with the lily pads and the four junipers standing sentry, one on each corner—how pleasant to wander here alone on a September day, lost in thought or maybe trying to memorize some lines of Tennyson, oblivious even to the bee sipping nectar noisily beside you as you walk down the "Dean's Walk" or in the "tunnel of gloom" under the overlapping trees near the western edge of the garden. The willows shake in the breeze, the fir trees wear their red berries like tiny rubies. And O ye flowers, so many of you, amaranth, delphinium, marigold, nasturtium, mum: I vow to buy a book and memorize all your names.

70

Armistice Day, 1970

The nurse comes in to check my wound and take my vitals but I don't know why she's here because it's November 11 and the war to end all wars ended fifty-two years ago today and I'm in England in 1970, a student at Clare College, Cambridge. The official hands me a folder full of papers. "Have a safe trip," she says. I am in the passenger seat of a car going to the American Cemetery three miles west of Cambridge. They are unveiling a plaque today at the grave of Peter Lehman, son of New York governor Herbert Lehman, one of the 3,812 servicemen buried or memorialized here, many of them casualties of the strategic air bombing of northwest Europe in World War II.

What explained the error perhaps was the strike of British postal workers (and the sympathy strike of telecommunication workers)—or maybe just bureaucratic sloppiness. The authorities wanted a family member present, if possible, but there was no budget for it, and the name Lehman on the Clare College roster caught someone's eye. I tried to explain, but the fact that I had the same surname as the deceased struck the organizers as reason enough for my being there. The senior tutor of my college summoned me to his office. These sorts of things happen, he said. You'll be doing us a favor. And, Mr. Lehman, be discreet.

It began to drizzle. I walked across the cemetery's great mall with its reflecting pools. From this vantage you could see the wide sweeping curve of the burial grounds, the concentric circles of graves that made this seem a piece of England that will forever be American. Minutes later, I found myself at the grave of Peter Lehman, fighter pilot, killed in action in World War II. Born in the Bronx, the valiant young man joined the Canadian Air Force in the early days of the conflict, before the United States entered the fray, and served in the US Air Force after declarations of war were made in December 1941. A member of the fabled Fourth Fighter Group stationed in England, he flew fifty-seven combat missions in Europe. He was an ace pilot. Perhaps the most celebrated of his exploits took place in February 1944. After attacking as many as twelve enemy aircraft to rescue a B-17, he downed two 190s before having his rudder shot away. On March 27, 1944, he flew in the attack on the Pau-Pont-Long aerodrome in France. The attack destroyed twenty-three enemy planes on the ground. Just four days later he died in his fighter plane. It was supposed to be a rest day, but he volunteered when a man who was scheduled to fly fell ill. The Distinguished Flying Cross, given for an exceptional act of heroism in an aerial flight, was awarded to him posthumously.

I lowered my head as everyone else did when the words on the plaque were recited. I thought: "The fear of the Lord is the beginning of all wisdom." Walking away I felt pride in my namesake's heroism.

Then they drove me back to Cambridge, where George Steiner, the resident polymath at Churchill College, was scheduled to deliver a lecture on "language, silence, and the sublime pain of being."

71

The Sublime Pain of Being

Not a day without pain. If not the neuropathy, the problems of adjusting to your prosthetic device, which sometimes malfunctions. The scar where they cut you open and the irritated skin surrounding the stoma. The seemingly interminable indigestion. These are unpleasant but banal. Only on some days do you feel the sublime pain of being alone in the universe. Like the experience of standing on a hotel room terrace in Miami during a hurricane watching the wind subdue the royal palms, taking them down, all the way down to the point where they are level with the ground; the storm howling in delight at its conquered foes—it puts the fear of the Lord in you. Back in September 2005 I was in Aventura on Florida's Atlantic coast when Hurricane Katrina made landfall there. The passengers aboard the aircraft two days later were as hushed as the audience hearing a certain four-and-a-half minute John Cage composition.

Most of the time the pain is physical, and you are reminded that your superbly functioning mind is imprisoned in your decaying body. Sometimes pain turns into rage. When Edward Said was dying of leukemia he told me he had become incredibly angry. With whom? "Oh, there's never a shortage of targets," he said.

This association of thoughts took place in the patient's mind as the technician pulled a switch and the machine wheeled the gurney into the cave where the body from the neck down would be photographed and X-rayed, with contrast, the dye shooting down his veins and arteries, and for a second he saw himself as the glass skeleton on the teacher's desk, with all his organs on display.

72

The Glass Skeleton

The boy frequented the Inwood branch of the New York Public Library and read more books than anyone else in the class. He was the first to identify all the parts in the glass skeleton on the teacher's desk. After school, he stood under a tree discussing baseball statistics, and the first-grade teacher walked by and went from being Miss Goodman to being Mrs. Sokolov. Miss Obendorf of the second grade became Mrs. Rosenblatt of the sixth. The Arden Street boys gathered to play punchball. As the youngest, Joel and David were team mascots assigned the task of choosing up sides. In 1957 Joel chose Harvey and David chose Harold and was thought to have got the better of the deal. Two years later Harold and his younger brother would go with their father to watch Floyd Patterson get knocked down seven times in one round by Ingemar Johansson.

Why was it so easy to remember the names of the managers of the National League teams in 1957? The boy learned a lot from comic books (Classics Illustrated) and the backs of bubble gum cards, and he had a good memory even then: he could identify the inventor of the reaper, the first man to go to the South Pole, John Paul Jones, Generals Grant and Lee, the rings of Saturn, and Joan of Arc. His father took him to the United Nations, his mother to Coney Island and to the Statue of Liberty, where both of them climbed the stairs all the way up to the top. His sister drew multicolored maps of Central and South America on oak tag and he brought them in and the teacher hung them on the bulletin board. Everyone else was older then, and all adults were expected to know the right answer, or at least directions home.

On a sunny Sunday afternoon in May 1957 he and his father sat in the stands in box seats ten rows behind Gil Hodges at first base as the Dodgers beat their archenemy the New York Giants, 5–3, at Ebbets Field. Duke Snider homered for the Dodgers, Ray Jablonski for the Giants. Pitching for the Dodgers that day was a local boy, who had played first base at Lafayette High and basketball at the University of Cincinnati—a Jewish "bonus baby" with a fantastic fastball, a lot of potential, but somewhat erratic results thus far in his Major League career: Sandy Koufax. The grass at Ebbets Field was the greenest the eight-year-old poet had ever seen. Clem Labine relieved Koufax in the eighth inning, and Snider made a shoestring catch to close out the game.

I was hooked. Vin (then Vince) Scully and Jerry Doggett broadcast the Dodger games that year, and the postgame radio show was co-hosted by Marty Glickman and Gussie Moran with a memorable jingle from Merkel Meats.* That is my main memory of the summer of 1957. Heartbreaking to fall in love with a team that would move to California at the end of that very season, taking the Giants along with them and resituating their old inter-borough rivalry to Los Angeles and San Francisco.

In 1957 I couldn't see the blackboard from the back of the classroom and I prayed every night that I wouldn't need eyeglasses. Prayer didn't work but it helped cushion the blow when it came.

---

* "Merkel meats are so good good good, / Taste and quality understood. / It's heard all over the neighborhood: / A great big 'mmmm' for Merkel."

And on October 4, 1957, the Soviets launched Sputnik. I went with my father and my sister to the roof of our apartment building to observe the sky. It was one of the really important dates of the twentieth century but sometimes overlooked, like the day in 1964 (January 11) when the Surgeon General's committee issued its report advising that smoking causes lung cancer.

73

Why Does the Bridge Not Progress?

Susan Sontag had it figured out. Diseases are metaphors that should not be used. Consumption is a romantic disease (Keats). Madness is a condition of genius and syphilis is the punishment for it (Nietzsche). Cancer: the disease of the loveless, the unhappy, the repressed "Miss Gee" in W. H. Auden's ballad, or any of the people seen at a distance from atop the Riesenrad in Vienna—insignificant, expendable, and easily replaced, as Harry Lime explains to his erstwhile buddy in *The Third Man*.

> *Soldiers and not slaves, prisoners and not soldiers. May I call your attention to Article Twenty-seven of the Geneva Convention? I happen to have a copy of it with me. For he's a jolly good fellow and so say all of us.*

"You can reframe your cancer," the social worker says. "You can choose wellness. Wellness is a positive choice. It is something every healthy cancer patient can achieve."

> *Two soldiers shot, the third drowned: to what end? Don't talk to me of rules. This is war, not a game of cricket. It's a matter of principle. If we give in now there'll be no end of it. That man is the worst commanding officer I have ever seen. Actually I think he's mad.*

"Do you know what you may be overlooking? Forgiveness. Forgiveness is the skeleton key to the temple door of your wellness. It is through forgiveness that you begin to heal. You start by letting yourself off the hook. Forgive your lungs, your pancreas, your bladder, your throat, your prostate, your testicles, your breasts, your ovaries, your liver, your cervix, your colon, your—you fill in the blank. Now feel the warmth of the glow of forgiveness."

You make me sick with your heroics—how to die like a gentleman
when the only important thing is how to live like a human being.
I must be off. The men are preparing some sort of entertainment.
"The King!"

"Have you expressed your gratitude today? Every healthy cancer patient of mine does five things every day, and exuding thankfulness is one of them. Thankfulness, because you are a guest on earth, a visitor, and because all time is a gift, and being here is a blessing that has been bestowed on you even in the darkest hour of treatment. Because you *are* blessed. And you *can* bless. Prayer is how you bless. Prayer and meditation lead to salvation."

He's gone mad, he's leading them right to it, our own man!
I was right, there is something going on.
Kill him! Kill him!
Kill him! Kill him!
"You!"
"You."
"What have I done?"
"Madness! Madness!"

74

Q & A

"When did you starting thinking of yourself as a writer?"

As a freshman in college I wrote poems almost every day. But I was also determined to become a good writer of prose and I thought I had the instincts of a good editor. In my senior year Paul Spike and I ate Szechuan food at Chuan-Hong on 106th Street and he generously asked me to join him as co-editor of the *Columbia Review*.

"How did you expect to earn a living?"

I taught full-time for five years, four of them at Hamilton College in upstate New York. The period from 1976 to 1980 occurred exactly a decade after my own college career and so it felt as if I had a second chance to go to college—this time from the point of view of a junior faculty member in a bucolic and peaceful setting as opposed to the rough-and-tumble of the big city in years of conflict and loathing. Hamilton was preppy in the L. L. Bean manner, while its sister institution, Kirkland, took pride in its offerings in modern dance and the theater arts. Opposites attract, and the two colleges merged in 1978. I had a ball. The students were only eight to twelve years younger than I, and fun to hang out with. So I guess I thought I would have an academic career.

In 1980, Archie Ammons arranged a postdoctoral fellowship at Cornell. Once I arrived in Ithaca, I never left. It was in Ithaca that I came to realize that a glorious future was behind me and I had better look for work in some other field than the English departments of American universities. To quit academe, to make it on my own as a writer, I had to reinvent myself. This was probably the most significant professional decision I ever made.

"Of what accomplishment are you proudest?"

When I turned forty, a friend asked me that question and I said, "Paying the rent." He looked bewildered but what the hell we clicked glasses and drank.

"Doesn't being the inventor of the *Best American Poetry* series thrust you right into the center of discourse where you are regarded as a gatekeeper and sometimes a leading member of the establishment?"

Oh, that's a load of crap. You know what Othello says before he stabs himself? "I have done the state some service, and they know't."

"What does that have to do with anything?"

I just like it. But to get back to your question, there is a certain burden of responsibility in sponsoring an annual anthology that calls itself *The Best American Poetry*. The editors take this responsibility very seriously.

"That sounds canned."

It has the virtue of being true. The book's objective is to serve poetry and poets, to make the case for the art, to acknowledge its audience and to enlarge it, and we have done this to the best of our ability from the start.

"You speak of academe with such skepticism and sometimes even contempt, though you teach and have taught, at least part-time, for the last twenty years."

I love teaching. But leaving academe when I did, refusing to go up the usual tenure ladder, made me feel free. As a journalist I didn't have to please anyone—except editors and copy editors and fact-checkers, who can be very exacting. My moneymaking activity was one thing and my poetry was another. This was liberating. My poetry did not have to do anything for me—it didn't have to get me a fancy teaching appointment or link me professionally with others of my generation. The whole burden was on my prose. Writing for *Newsweek* was akin to being an educator, bringing word to the public of some cultural event they should know about. And doing it on deadline. I learned how to write clearly and how to write fast, and these abilities are invaluable.

"A former student of yours said that you were a natural as a lecturer."

That's very nice to hear. Teaching is harder than it looks. It took me a long time to learn how to manage an assortment of people into a cohesive group where everyone can speak freely without fear of ridicule or contempt and the atmosphere is, by semester's end, almost joyous as we revel in having had this shared experience.

"Did you enjoy the life of the campus poet?"

Living in a comic academic novel is amusing, especially if the author is Mary McCarthy, Randall Jarrell, or Kingsley Amis. A senior professor on the Cornell faculty, now deceased, once told me he was writing poems and sending them out. But, he said, he kept getting rejection letters that were remarkably ambiguous. He couldn't figure them out. Would I come to the office and take a look? He had collected all the rejection letters. It turned out that all of them were form letters. The usual thing: not right for our pages, but we thank you for thinking of us. There was no proof that any human being had thought twice about them. I looked at the senior professor and could tell that he wasn't putting me on.

At my first faculty meeting at Hamilton College, back in 1976, they were arguing about the librarians. Should they be invited to faculty meetings and if so, should they be entitled to vote? Should they be seated separately? "Why don't you invite them?" I said with poker face. "After one meeting, they may not want to come back." The chairman of the English department was not amused. He called me into his office. He was a wonderful example of the freckle-faced country club Harvard alum, a bright, good-natured guy who ends up divorcing his beautiful, alcoholic wife and pairing off with the cute Jewish divorcee in the admissions office. At least the curriculum made sense: *Beowulf,* Chaucer, *Sir Gawain and the Green Knight*, Sir Thomas Wyatt, Spenser, Marlowe, Shakespeare, Milton, the Metaphysicals, Ben Jonson, Swift, "The Rape of the Lock," Gray's "Elegy," Samuel Johnson, Christopher Smart. That was English 200. How wonderful to teach "Lycidas" or "A Modest Proposal." And even freshman English, the most painful of all pedagogic duties, had a departmentally chosen reading list that in my time routinely included works by Homer, Sophocles, Plato, Virgil, Dante, Shakespeare, Voltaire, Goethe, Jane Austen, Stendhal, Dostoyevsky, Tolstoy, Ibsen, Freud, Conrad, and Shaw. You had to give them that, the proud traditionalists on the faculty at Hamilton back then: they believed in what they were teaching.

75

Ludlowville, 1981

B eing sick gives a man the gift of speech. He doesn't necessarily use it wisely, but use it he does.

Waking up some days reminds me of waking up in Ludlowville, thirty-three years old, wondering: How did I get here? Not in a philosophical sense, not in the spirit of Bertrand Russell convinced that we have no real proof that the world existed before we woke up, let alone before we were born.

No: How did I get to this dead end?

Ludlowville, a little hamlet about seven miles north of Ithaca on the east bank of Cayuga Lake, where I was down and out, was a good place to spend your wilderness years. If you measure happiness by how few people you need to be in contact with, Ludlowville was heaven.

In 1981 I didn't get the job I thought I wanted and I spent my birthday afternoon hiding on a shady ledge high above a gorge in the former Enfield Glen, now Upper Treman State Park. Later that day Stefanie and I drove to Ludlowville and rented the first house we saw. I liked the black shutters and the white Doric columns up front. The house was uninsulated and we used kerosene heaters and a woodstove to heat the place when summer faded away. You could get a standard cord of wood dumped in your backyard for $80 if you were willing to stack it yourself. Winter was a trial, and it began promptly on the first of November. But summer was a bounty of splendor, of "foison": the beauty of radishes, beets, and berries. Melons, white peaches, plums, apricots, white nectarines. Just-picked corn on the cob fresh off the shuck, no need to boil. Tomatoes in the garden like poppies in a field. In fall, the many varieties of apple. The rush of water overcoming the rock of resistance where brook widens into stream, which you trace to a waterfall in the undiscovered woods. You take off your clothes in reverence.

In 1981 Tom Kheel explained supply-side economics to me. I'm not sure I got it but I listened as he drove us in his Toyota pickup truck to Syracuse where we watched the Blue Jays' Triple-A team take on Columbus. Tom owned a bar, the Dugout, with great Yankees photographs, pennants, and autographed baseballs in his back room. It was a place where partygoers from Ithaca College came with fake IDs and carried on flirtations or fistfights. Tom had to hire a bouncer. He pitched for a local softball team and tutored me on how to use small-claims court to advantage.

On a hot July day in Ludlowville in 1981 I went to the woods, sat on a rock as the water streamed past me, and these words came to my mind: "Alas, what boots it with uncessant care / To tend the homely slighted shepherd's trade?" Yes, I thought. That just about sums it up.

In 1981 I took a daily walk into the woods and noticed that Tom's dog Bruno, a red coon hound, was coming along with me. He was my walking partner thereafter. Bruno was Ludlowville.

76

Bio Note (Alt.)

David Lehman was born in New York City in 1948, the son of Jewish refugees from Hitler's Europe. His family lived in an apartment in Washington Heights, a few blocks away from the northernmost entrance of Fort Tryon Park, near Dyckman Street, the heart of Inwood, with its two movie theaters, two kosher delis, two bakeries, two newsstands, and two Chinese restaurants. His mother was cheerful, gregarious. His father—serious, hardworking, disciplined, orderly—chewed gum (Chiclets) because chewing gum was American; he liked it when little David, asked about his father's occupation, answered, he's "a businessman."

Raised as an Orthodox Jew, educated at a yeshiva through grade school, Lehman attended Stuyvesant High School, did well at history and math, and held a part-time after-school job making minimum wage ($1.40 an hour) as a shipping clerk for a company that manufactured and distributed tachometers and other electrical devices. He learned how to use a box cutter, how to pack boxes, when to use excelsior, which parcels went to Railway Express or UPS and which had to be lugged to the post office, where he added to his collection of mint plate blocks of four. He got to lock up the office on the day of the big blackout on November 9, 1965. It was rush hour. At Chambers Street he got into the A train, found a seat, started reading a book (*USA* by John Dos Passos). The train stopped shy of the West Fourth Street station. Everyone was quiet for the first thirty minutes. A man broke the silence, and soon this crowd of strangers cohered into a group, making wisecracks, buddying up, laughing it off. After four hours, the straphangers walked along the subway tracks when it was ascertained that there was no longer any danger of electrocution. Emerging onto Eighth Street and Sixth Avenue, people celebrated as if it were New Year's. Someone had a car and asked if anyone needed a ride to the George Washington Bridge and he got in. At 181st Street and Broadway he caught the Broadway bus and was not charged a fare. He got out at Nagle Avenue and was treated like a hero by his mother when she heard his key in the lock at eleven o'clock.

The day he got into Columbia was the happiest day in his life. At Columbia he reviewed the occasional Broadway play for the *Columbia Daily Spectator*, played tennis, and swam the 200-meter breaststroke. He fell in love, had his heart broken, went to bed with a girl and woke up a different man. He shared digs with Carlton, who changed his name to Jamal and explained the allure of John Coltrane, "the Malcolm X of jazz." He listened to "Giant Steps" and got totally into jazz. Majoring in history, he wrote a thesis on the retired Jackie Robinson's columns for the *New York Post*, then a liberal tabloid, and his friendship with New York governor Nelson Rockefeller. Awarded the Kellett Fellowship for two years of study at Cambridge, he stayed in Europe for a third year, in Paris mostly. A telegram summoned him home. At JFK he learned from his uncle Raymond that his father had died that day.

It was time to curb his wanderlust. He now had to provide for his widowed mother and younger siblings. Through Raymond Lehman's influence, he got into an executive training program at Merrill Lynch, did well, worked there, got a better job with E. F. Hutton, impressed the boss with his stock-picking skills, and moved on to work for the legendary Peter Lynch, who ran the Fidelity Magellan Fund in its heyday. In 1990 he signed on as a senior analyst for Michael Price's Mutual Series. In the 1990s he did well—hell, everybody did well—and he made smart side bets on IBM (at fire-sale prices in 1993), Coke, Gillette, Atlantic Richfield, Warner-Lambert, Pfizer, and American Express. He laid down a pile on Cisco, EMC, Microsoft, and Intel when the going was good and took his chips off the table in January 2000, just a few months before the dot-com bubble burst.

After 9/11, he decided that the twentieth century—a foreshortened century, lasting only eighty-seven years, with three global wars, one of them cold—had ended. (By contrast, the nineteenth century lasted ninety-nine years, from Waterloo in 1815 to Sarajevo in 1914.) He liquidated all his holdings except for a regional bank and some water utilities, put most of the dough in treasuries and savings accounts, and moved to a little hamlet in the Finger Lakes. He persuaded the woman he had been dating to join him and he married her. There was more than enough money for them to live on comfortably. The house they lived in backed on a sloping green yard. Beyond it a stream ran, and across the stream was a wooded hill. Four dogs kept him company on his romps in the woods. His mother came to visit, took a look at the rustic quarters, and described the place as *"wo die Teufel gute Nacht sagt."**

It was here that he wrote his acclaimed book on how Western culture has assimilated the theories of Sigmund Freud, the maligning of the man notwithstanding. *Freud from Nietzsche to Trilling* was nominated for the Bonker Prize in 2015. His wife was active in the local farmers' market and wrote a syndicated column that locavores loved. The couple had a baby grand and whiled away some enchanted evenings singing old favorites, "Blue Room" and "Let's Fall in Love," "Tea for Two" and "Someone to Watch Over Me."

---

* "Where the devil says good night."

77

Wedding Ceremony

In 2005, Harold Arlen's centenary, I read Robert Pinsky's book on King David and thought I could write a book for the same series of books on Jewish themes. It would be either on five lyricists (Hart, Gershwin, Fields, Harburg, Cahn) or maybe on a single composer, Arlen or Richard Rodgers.

At Stacey's instigation I started making collages and postcard-sized paintings. JA liked the one I made for him after we visited the Ashbery Farms in Sodus, New York, where John grew up.

At the wedding ceremony Stacey quoted "Time After Time" (music Jule Styne, lyrics Sammy Cahn) and I quoted "That Old Black Magic" (music Harold Arlen, lyrics Johnny Mercer). It was the sixteenth of August, two days before her birthday. Ron Leifer was my witness. I forget the judge's name but she was very sweet.

The wedding party at 70 Jane was unforgettable, thank you Bill and Jay.

That was the year we went to Poland. "Tell no Polish jokes," Billy Collins advised. "I don't know Polish," I said.

When we got back I told Ashbery about the torn bedsheets in our bedroom in Warsaw and he said "tear sheets" in his deadpan way.

At the station in Poznan I spilled coffee on my white shirt and grimaced. Paweł Marcinkiewicz, my poet friend, said, "Relax. Now you look Polish." Waiting for the train he instructed me to stand in the middle of the platform, because, he pointed, sometimes the train stops there (fifty feet to the left) and sometimes it stops there (fifty feet the other way). It arrived fifty feet to our left. We ran, I tripped over the straps of my carry-on, flew into the air, landed on my knees, and reached the train breathless, bloody. As the train started pulling out of the station, Paweł said, "Now you look even more Polish."

Poland of dreams, Poland of death. We arrived in Lodz and the man at the train station said you must want to see the Jewish cemetery. So we drove there, our suitcases in the boot, but it was closed. Undeterred our guide drove us to the Holocaust memorial museum, outside which young people stood and smoked. It seemed to be in the shape of an oven with a thin stream of smoke drifting upward from the center. After you walked down the corridor past the photographs of people killed in the camps you emerged in an open space. There was a cattle car there, one they had used to transport Jews to Auschwitz. The doors were wide open. I declined an invitation to check out the inside of the car. "I might never get out," I said to our host, who laughed but didn't quite get my point.

Our host from the university took us to the Jewish theme restaurant in Lodz named Anatewka. When you enter, you're greeted by a life-sized doll of a Hassidic man in a prayer shawl. The walls are lined with paint-by-number portraits of distinguished-looking rabbis. We dined on borscht, chopped liver, and "Goose Goulash in Jewish Sauce."[*]

When you leave Anatewka, they give you, as a memento of the occasion, a little plastic figure of a long-nosed Jew with *peyyot* or

---

[*] You can look it up: https://www.tripadvisor.com/ShowUserReviews-g274837-d749996-r596588315-Anatewka-Lodz_Lodz_Province_Central_Poland.html.

a rebbe with a prayer shawl holding a worthless coin, the zloty equivalent of a penny. I was reminded of Hitler's goal of killing the Jews then making a museum devoted to this lost people.

Next to the sculpture of Artur Rubinstein and his piano I understood it for the first time. It was a miracle. You could have anti-Semitism without Jews. You didn't even need Jews!

78

Moscow, 2007

In Moscow in October 2007. Stacey and I stayed at the Peking Hotel in Mayakovsky Square, dominated by a statue of the poet.

"You see, the Russians build statues of their great poets," the scholar Mikoyan said.

"But not until they have driven them to commit suicide," I countered.

"That was the Soviets," he said. "Not the Russians."

The October Revolution had taken place exactly ninety years ago this week but nothing in Moscow told you it was an important anniversary.

A Russian novelist took me to breakfast and ordered eggs, bacon, sausage, pancakes for herself. For me she ordered pickles and jam—and nothing else. "But they are the house specialties," she said. I asked her whether she could write while drinking, and she said, "My dear David, if you could not write when you drink, there would be no such thing as Russian literature." That night I went shot for shot with a poet from Georgia and I got drunk and Stacey got mad even though I would have insulted his honor—and let down the American side—had I refused to join him.

Russian proverbs. Vodka was the usual subject. Stalin said, "If the enemy won't surrender, we will utterly consume him," and the saying had it that "vodka is our enemy, so we must utterly consume it." When saying yes to the offer of a glass, you might say, "Certainly. After all, the owl is the only creature that doesn't drink, if only because she sleeps in the daytime and the stores are closed at night."

Allowing for differences in language, custom, culture, race, and national identity, the people in the Moscow subway looked pretty much like the people riding the New York subway at rush hour on a winter morning. Curious, suspicious, harried, sleepy. Across the street from the Kremlin, the lines at McDonald's stretched around the corner. Never was I happier to see a McDonald's.

The casino on the ground floor of the Peking Hotel was like casinos everywhere, without windows or clocks. Street signs on the wall featured the misspelled names of New York locales: Harlem, Broadway, Wall Street. The café on the other side of the lobby was a convenient hangout for local harlots, who rang the doorbell of single male residents at two in the morning. It was here that I met Suslov. Suslov chain-smoked unfiltered cigarettes. Between great puffs of white smoke he volunteered that he remained a believer in Marxist theory. Didn't the sorry fate of the Bolshevik Revolution refute it? "What Lenin and the party did wasn't really Marxism," Suslov said. I thought but didn't say that there are professors of literature in North America who say the same thing about the Russians and Marxism. *They didn't really try it.*

Later that week, after a tour of the permanent exhibit at the Mayakovsky Museum, a man wearing a yellow vest offered me a glass of horseradish-flavored vodka. I drank it. Then another. "I heard that Suslov has been arrested," he said casually. The toilet in the Mayakovsky Museum didn't flush properly and there was no paper other than the Kleenex I had in my pocket. Exiting from the back door, I felt guilty and unclean when I reached the street. Talk about widening income inequality—the Russians have us beat in that department.

The car had left without me. I flagged down the driver of a black car and bribed him extra to take me back to the hotel.

"You forget something," he said in heavily accented English, handing me an old and worn manila envelope. Then he drove off. I shoved it into my briefcase and went up to the room before opening it. Inside was the manuscript of *The Counterfeiters*—not a translation of André Gide's novel but a fantasia on it embedded in a narrative about a man who commits gratuitous crimes.

It would take me months of sustained effort to decode it after my friend Andrey translated it for me.

79

Group Therapy

Geiger, the cancer psychologist, invites me to join his support group of bladder cancer patients who meet once a month to talk and to "reach out for support." I know I'm going to hate it, but I go.

Each of us has to imagine a place of our own to which we can retreat when we need to withdraw into our own minds. When we need to shut out the rest of the world. We are asked to describe the place as well as we can. Comes my turn and I summon up the image of a trailer in the wilderness, six or seven dogs of different breeds running around the place, a rooster, hens. It is summer. There are tires, maybe a score of them, along the side of the driveway, and marijuana plants in the back.

80

Fort Tryon Park

I enjoy my dreams once I wake up and realize they're not true. These days, as I lie in bed exhausted after walking a mere two or three city blocks, my dreams are in American English with German subtitles or Hebrew with English subtitles or sometimes they are French movies with subtitles that leave out half the dialogue. The lead actor plays a boy with his share of imaginary friends who convened in Fort Tryon Park until another boy from school joined him and exposed the fraud. The boy could imitate an eagle. In the park there were caves, secret silver mines, rare minerals, and the knowledge that the Revolutionary War was fought here in the heights of this park where stood George Washington himself, in whose honor the bridge bearing his name leads west from 179th Street. The boy memorized the phone numbers of friends and called stockbrokers to discuss transactions though he was not yet twelve years old. He made his own postage stamps and tried using them until the postman returned the letters to his mother and explained the situation. He collected stamps because his father did. He rooted for the Dodgers because his cousin Johnny did. His cousin didn't have a TV but he slept over and they listened to *The Lone Ranger* on the radio. Your childhood is the part of you to which you naturally return at the end.

That, and the endless dialogue about God and faith.

81

A Fine Invention

The moment when you realize that death is not an abstraction. When does it happen? "When the father dies," Freud says. Freud and I have had many conversations about my dreams. Sometimes he analyzes them, sometimes we talk as we walk on city streets or paths in Buttermilk Falls State Park. We devoted an entire day to the principle that life is a preparation for death, for death is the aim of life. He explained why the third in any feminine series stood for death: Aphrodite, Cinderella, Cordelia, the third casket in *The Merchant of Venice*. I handed him a twenty to settle a wager when the youngest daughter on *Downton Abbey* died.

A. J. Ayer on the meaning of life: God is a "useful myth," a view so modest there seems little point in disputing it. "There is, indeed, no ground for thinking that human life in general serves any ulterior purpose but this is no bar to a man's finding satisfaction in many of the activities which make up his life." That "but" clause sounds a trifle halfhearted, don't you think?

W. H. Auden said the trick of living in New York City lay in crossing the street against the light. I say, "If I didn't believe in God, I wouldn't be able to cross a New York street even when the light is green." You say it's the green light that keeps me safe, and the assumption of sanity based on collective self-interest that governs motorists and makes them hit the brakes when the light turns red. Science has made religion obsolete and we are an irreversibly secular society. Why do you think the radical Islamists are so pissed off?

"Faith is a fine invention," Emily Dickinson wrote. But, she added, in an emergency "microscopes are more prudent." This from Emily, who lives in the afterlife.

Theology is not a prudent motorist. Faith makes you turn right at the corner of Aquinas and Pascal, a street leading to a cul-de-sac. There is no use resorting to logic as you did in the old days when (you boasted) any atheist could win a logical argument against the existence of God. Well, maybe, but that atheist wasn't on his deathbed at the time, or in a trench in Flanders, avoiding three on a match when the fellows lighted their fags because a light lasting that long could get you killed. As an old man, the English philosopher Antony Flew found God after spending a lifetime disproving His existence. Flew, once known in Oxbridge circles as "the world's most notorious atheist," declared that there is a God with a capital G after all, an Aristotelian God who doesn't intervene in the universe. The octogenarian Flew was co-author of *There Is a God*, though when interviewed on the subject he would draw a blank and talk candidly about his memory loss.

JA and I were discussing the possible existence of God. He believed in God, he said. "But how would you define it?" I mentioned Anselm's ontological argument. If God is that than which nothing greater can be or be conceived, there must be a God. But that is just a cover for the semantic proof—that is, God as a concept must exist since we have the word "God," a weak argument that plays down the element of faith.

I said: "You know how in Alcoholics Anonymous they have to begin by acknowledging a power in the universe greater than the self?"

"Yes," John said dryly. "Alcohol."

82

Identity Theft

David A. Lehman (Washington and Lee, '99) is the global head of real estate finance at Goldman Sachs. Prior to assuming his role in the Investment Banking Division, David was co-head of mortgage trading in the Securities Division. He joined Goldman Sachs in 2004 as a vice president and was named managing director in 2006 and partner in 2008. Testifying before Congress regarding the financial crisis of 2008–9, he used the phrase "sourced from the Street" and was asked to explain it. He said, "The phrase is accurate because, even though all the assets were acquired from the Goldman ABS Desk, Goldman is a part of 'the Street.'"

David Lehman graduated from Loyola Law School. Since 2002 he has been Deputy Executive Director and General Counsel of the National Rifle Association's Institute for Legislative Action, the lobbying arm of the NRA. "If somebody wants to use [an assault weapon] to protect their family, protect their home, or if they want to engage in target shooting and competitive shooting, then they ought to have the right to do that," Mr. Lehman said, "if they're a law-abiding citizen and all that. We feel that it's much more important to go after the criminal than to go after the gun." Mr. Lehman said it's ludicrous that gun makers should "be liable for the unforeseeable acts of criminals."

David Lehman works for NASA. He confirmed that NASA has named the site where twin agency spacecraft impacted the moon Monday in honor of the late astronaut Sally K. Ride, who was America's first woman in space and a member of the probe's mission team. The impact marked a successful end to GRAIL, NASA's lunar mission to carry cameras fully dedicated to education and public outreach. "Ebb fired its engines for 4 minutes, 3 seconds and Flow fired its for 5 minutes, 7 seconds," said Lehman, GRAIL project manager at NASA's Jet Propulsion Laboratory (JPL) in Pasadena, Calif. "It was one final important set of data from a mission that was filled with great science and engineering data."

David Lehman is chairman of Dominion Systems, a London-based firm that formerly manufactured gas chambers, electric chairs, and other execution equipment for state-sponsored use and now makes limited-edition replicas for collectors and museums.

David Lehman built a twenty-foot wooden speedboat in the basement of his parents' house in Lansing, New York. It took the happily married, self-employed carpenter three years to complete the project with the assistance of "a bunch of guys who wanted [to take part] in the journey."

Dave Lehman, 23, and his associate, George Bailey, 22, attempted to steal a four-wheeler from a home on Brickyard Hill Road early Thursday morning. When the victim confronted the suspects, they fled. Deputies responded and apprehended the suspects within minutes. They were taken to the Cayuga County Jail on a preliminary charge of burglary.

David J. Lehman was born in Dallas, Texas, on April 5, 1947. A petty officer second class for the United States Navy during the Vietnam War, he died on December 14, 1968, at the age of 21 in Hau Nghia, a victim of small arms fire.

83

A Routine Visit

First you wait. Then your name is called. You must confirm it and provide your birth date. Then your vitals are taken. 98.1, 131 over 73, very good. Then you wait. Then you repeat steps one through three. Then your name is called. Then she escorts you to an exam room. Then you wait. Then she asks you for your name and birth date. Then the doctor's intern (or "fellow," as they're called in this medical hierarchy) comes in, listens to your heart and lungs, feels your stomach and legs, asks whether you feel pain or nausea or have had a fever or chills or get winded after climbing a flight of steps. The intern went to Princeton, Michigan, and Johns Hopkins. Then you wait. The doctor enters and tells you the results of the scan, which indicate that you fractured two ribs recently. Somehow this happened without your knowing it. Then Jenny enters, draws the curtain, masks herself, masks you, draws blood from your port, and flushes it. Then you can go.

The next day you report to the neurology specialist. You repeat steps one through three as above. Then you fill out some forms. Then you wait. Then the nurse escorts you to the examination room. The expensive Dr. Reich, first name Frank I believe, wears a white dress shirt, no tie, tasseled shoes, and gets right down to business. "On a scale from one to ten how much pain are you having?" "Eight." A Leonard Bernstein lookalike, he is stooped over. He needs knee replacement surgery, he says. He tells you he has put it off for a year. Then he asks you the same question he asked you when he entered the room, file in hand. "On a scale from one to ten how much pain are you having?" "Eight." When his back is turned you lower your voice and say, "Maybe you need a hearing aid." "What?" "I said eight," you say. Then he writes something down. Then you wait. Then he looks up. "On a scale from one to ten how much pain are you having?" He lowers his head, you lower your voice and whisper, "Hearing aid." "What?" "Eight." Then he leaves the room. Then you get dressed. Then you can go.

84

Doctor Jew

This is what you need to know: "operation" is now "procedure," and "pain" is now "discomfort." We don't say "remission." We say "no evidence of disease" or "no new suspicious findings," which doesn't mean that there's no cancer, just that if there is any, we can't see it. It is always understood to be a temporary condition. Okay? "No problem."

"When we said you'll feel better in six months, that's doctor speak for a year," Dr. Castle confided.

"Does that ratio apply to all prognosticative medical statements?"

"Well, no, I wouldn't go that far. People think science is infallible. It isn't. It's just educated guesswork based on empirically verifiable evidence and a history of medical precedents. Fighting disease is like working in the dark. For most people the darkness is total. The best we can do is to bring a flashlight along."

Can't eat anything except toast with jam, fig jam or raspberry jam or apricot jam, or a piece of dark chocolate. Can't drink anything except a cup of unsweetened tea, Assam or English Breakfast, and maybe later in the day a mug of fruit tea—they have a kind called "Blue Eyes" at McNulty's, so naturally that's the one I buy when Glen and the dogs and I walk to McNulty's. There are days when I can hardly negotiate the space between the apartment and the street. But I can write. And I can listen. And sometimes I can even hear the music of the spheres when Mahler's First or Tchaikovsky's Fifth Symphony is on satellite radio.

The steady diet of daytime television to which the convalescing patient is condemned will embitter any heart. The news is full of the bickering of politicians and their apologists and the pundits with trumped-up gravitas, masters of instant analysis whose predictions are always wrong. And the commercials have a cast of talking animals, dumb dads, super moms, gullible old people, vain young women, men who need back surgery, women who wish to preserve their dignity though they are martyrs to constipation and leakage, disembodied voices hawking reverse mortgages and gold coins, the voice of Don Draper hawking a Mercedes, the deep baritone voice touting real American beer as opposed to the effeminate pumpkin ale the high-end microbreweries are producing, local car dealers who think they're comedians, unfunny comedians selling the best light beer you've ever tasted, the enthusiastic inventor of the National Sleep Foundation's pillow of the year, a two-for-one deal and we'll throw in the shipping. Free; all you have to pay is a separate fee. In one car insurance spot "you totaled your car" or "tapped one little fender" and are righteously pissed off at your current insurer.

There is one commercial I genuinely like. An attractive couple is walking toward their house. She's wearing a mauve top; he's in a sport jacket and what look to be corduroy trousers. "I hope we've found a buyer for the house," she says. "Me too," he replies. But when they enter the house, "What are the neighbors doing here?" The real estate agent is isolated in the kitchen, shrugging her shoulders helplessly, and the neighbors, including a black man and his daughter and a white couple with their son—are occupying the house's armchairs and couches, and helping themselves to food from the kitchen, because, as the kids tell the dads, the cable provider and Internet outlet used by these fortunate folks is so superior to anything the neighbors have. It's "crazy fast," the boy exclaims. You can do more things on more devices in a single household with unlimited Wi-Fi everywhere. "Cool," says the dad. But my thoughts are with the couple who are trying to sell their house. What's their story? Why are they moving? Have they been married for a long time? Do they have kids? Do they still make love twice a week? And how will they tactfully get these obnoxious freeloaders out of the house?

Speaking of neighbors, the movie Stacey and I watched last night was *Gran Torino* (2008), directed by Clint Eastwood and starring Eastwood as a cranky bigoted septuagenarian monument to self-reliance who defiantly smokes cigarettes though he coughs up blood. Virtually all of Eastwood's neighbors are Asian and he uses a whole range of negative stereotypes and derogatory phrases—from "slopes" to "Charlie Chan"—in his encounters with them. But as is the way of such films, he becomes fond of a particular young Asian man and his sister, who are threatened by a gang of doped-up ne'er-do-wells, also Asian, with too many guns and too few brains. The movie is about the adjustment Eastwood's character makes upon finding, for example, that his regular doctor is gone and there is an Asian woman in his place. "Where's Dr. Feldman?" he asks. "He retired three years ago," she says. "I'm Dr. Chu." Eastwood scowls. And of course I heard "Dr. Jew," as if to underscore the point that the Asians are the new Jews—discriminated against because they are perceived to value education, a work ethic, ambition, good behavior, a sense of the rights and duties of citizenship. And of course Clint Eastwood turns out to be a good neighbor.

In San Francisco's Chinatown the smart set goes to Mister Jiu's where the cooking is overseen by Chinese American chef Brandon Jew. Immigration officials spelled it that way, Jew says. Foodies consider it a fun place, with excellent vegetables and a dressy crowd.

85

"Except for the cancer . . ."

"Don't fade into the sheets," Dr. Borodin says. It's a line I've heard before. It means I must get exercise if I want to recover. "Exercise and water are your medicines now."

I hiccupped for six straight hours. They phoned in a prescription for a muscle relaxant and it stopped right away. The entrepreneur in me thought: A good pre-massage cocktail consisting of muscle relaxant, truth serum, sexual stimulant, and vodka could sell millions.

So I start a prose poem: "As an ex-soldier returns to the postwar rubble in Berlin expecting to see what's left of the building in which he grew up playing with his cousins, so I visit you, my life."

Then I draft a novel. It begins: "'Except for the cancer, you're in excellent health,' the doctor said." What's the plot? An elderly professor of literature is diagnosed with cancer. He goes through all the indignities of chemotherapy and radical surgery. To pass the time he writes a roman à clef called *The Inferno* about treacherous colleagues he has known. The Inferno is the name of an air-conditioned museum to which the ailing man gains entrance through the intercession of two angels disguised as recent Barnard alums, Beth Hayes and Tess Zion. Inside the museum he encounters the effigies of Peter Rubella, heir to the German measles fortune; Polly Tzei, advocate of "preemptive censorship"; and Lois Menard, the Borges scholar and author of *In Praise of Plagiarism*, and her partner, Leon Elson, the Arthur Dimmesdale Professor of Serial Adultery, who has written a new book on *The Scarlet Letter* and dedicated it to his wife.

On television the host with the British accent asks a financial analyst about macroeconomic conditions given the headline risk in Europe, and the analyst says, "I'm agnostic about that," meaning he doesn't have an opinion one way or another. It's not that he's indifferent to the worrisome trend. It's that he doesn't know one way or the other, and it doesn't really matter. Sort of turns Pascal on his head, doesn't it? I mean today most people are wagering that God doesn't exist—if they think about it at all. That's the default position. Whereas Pascal thought that if you reduced it to a gamble, the smart money would go with God just in case.

How hard it is to walk one hundred years—I mean one hundred yards!—and I, an all-time speed walking champ with a determined frown on my face.

86

The Heart Knows

The heart may have its reasons but
the overcoat knows what it knows and
keeps the knowledge up its sleeves
or pocketed with torn theater stubs:
the hat on the rack longs for the head
uneasy on the pillow, the scarf recalls
the skater in the wind of his momentum,
and the black leather gloves retain
the shape of the fingers that clutched
the straps on the bus that connects
the city from one river to the other.

87

A Black Dress

I have a wound in my right side, a wound the size of a bullet hole. "We call it 'meat red,'" the nurse said. "It's like the inside of your mouth." For months I ignored it. Now I look at it incessantly. I feel it to make sure it's still there, like an aching tooth. A gaping red bullet hole, bigger than you'd think a bullet hole would be. I was shot, by whom I don't remember, in a quarrel over something insignificant, a pouch of wine, the way his woman looked at me in the bar. There my body lies, at the base of an enormous sycamore. I can see it clearly though I am standing miles away on the roof of a cabin using high-powered binoculars. In my professional life I continue just as before except for the red bullet hole in my red side, which is concealed by shirt and sweater. I weigh twenty-five pounds less but otherwise look pretty much the same. A little paler. Several battlefields ago I discarded the medals, the ribbons, the uniform. What good would they do me now? And then I realized that I am a ghost in a suit and tie.

That night I thought it through, sentence by sentence, an essay on the progression from sexual desire to love to marriage to divorce in America, how one thing leads to another with the inevitability of a loss in a baseball game when your team has a three-run lead in the seventh inning but your pitcher has walked the bases loaded and there's a pitching change and the other team capitalizes with a grand-slam home run and you're playing in their ballpark, enemy territory, sixty thousand cheering fans, and now it's the top of the eighth inning and the guy sitting next to you is your own father in a pensive mood, looking backward, his arm around you, reassuring you that your future won't be like that. He quotes Yogi Berra: "If I had to do it over, I'd do it over."

Meanwhile my wife visited a new therapist, who took one look at her and said: "You're wearing a black dress. Don't you know that black means death?" "But you're also wearing a black dress," my wife replied.

88

Heisenberg as Hero

I'll try anything. Nin's friend Sarah, my skillful acupuncturist, recommends taking three tablets of Resilience twenty minutes after breakfast, another three one hour before dinner, plus three tablets of Move Mountains twice daily, it doesn't matter when.

"What about maitake and turmeric?"

"You can't go wrong with maitake and turmeric."

Meanwhile, I wonder whether the ideal viewer of *Breaking Bad* is, as I am, a cancer patient in chemo with a son who suffers from cerebral palsy. I like Heisenberg as our hero's code name. And the apprentice chemist's corny recitation of Whitman's "When I Heard the Learned Astronomer," the poem that serves as the final clue to the drug lord's identity. And the photo of Elizabeth Bishop on the wall of a young woman, the landlord's daughter, who dies of a heroin overdose as a result of which her despondent dad, an air traffic controller, makes an error at work causing the worst plane wreck in Albuquerque history. Another episode ends with Skyler telling her husband, "I fucked Ted."

The year 1912, when the *Titanic* sank and the aristocracy was on the verge of killing itself off in a senseless war, is considered the best period to set a novel or a movie. I can see that and was a sucker for the first seasons of *Downton Abbey*, which I stopped watching when the showrunner shamelessly ripped off the scene in *Mrs. Miniver* in which the old dowager (Dame May Whitty), who usually awards herself the prize for the best rose at the annual flower show, decides to be magnanimous for once and declares the unassuming Henry Travers to be the winner. In the following scene, the Germans attack and Teresa Wright takes a bullet and Greer Garson comforts her, but we know she's going to die.

My hair has grown back. When people ask, I lie and say I feel a little better every day. I say there are three terrible lingering side effects but I don't say what they are. And sometimes I say for every two steps forward I need to move one step back when the reverse ratio comes closer to the fact.

89

Cheers!

The best commercial in Super Bowl 50 has a scowling Helen Mirren at a bar, with a huge hamburger, fries, and a bottle of beer in front of her. She scolds the viewer on the evils of drunk driving. Then she picks up a Budweiser and says, "Cheers!"

The lawyer preparing my revised will, Eric Kinsler by name, went to Columbia, just as I did, but twenty-five years later. The reading list still consisted (he tells me) of "dead white males."

"I wouldn't use that phrase," I said.

"Why not?"

"Because two of those terms apply to me and the third isn't very far away."

Both of us smiled to show there were no hard feelings. Then he said, "Relax, dude. You're not a white male. You're Jewish."

On the other hand, my friend Charlene complimented me the other day on being "woke" ahead of the curve.

90

Walter Lehmann

Among my father's cousins, Walter Lehmann was exceptional in four ways: he kept the double *n*'s at the end of his surname; after escaping from Nazi Germany, he settled in Australia rather than in England or the United States; he wrote poetry; and he was a purely fictional character, a persona and a pseudonym adopted by Gwen Harwood (1920–1995), an estimable Australian poet.

Married to a professor of linguistics at the University of Tasmania, Harwood was a lifelong student of Wittgenstein. She adopted other masks besides Walter Lehmann. "I like disguises," she said. "I like beards and wigs." But there was more to it than an attraction to the paraphernalia of masquerade. It was an example of practical feminism—a demonstration that a poem about a woman would have a chance to win the enthusiasm of an editor only if he thought a man had written it. It was also a fruitful way to question the concepts of identity and gender.

Harwood adopted the identity of Walter Lehmann most memorably in 1961, when she hoaxed the poetically conservative editor of the prestigious Sydney-based literary journal *The Bulletin*. Walter Lehmann wrote "A Kitchen Poem," a moving and much-lauded poem that explores the life of a mother and housewife from the female point of view. Gwen Harwood was convinced that "A Kitchen Poem" would not have been published under her own name because of the editor's gender bias, and so, as Walter Lehmann, she followed up with two acrostic sonnets that appeared in a subsequent issue of *The Bulletin*. There was egg on the venerable editor's face when Harwood pointed out that the first letters of the sonnets' lines, read vertically, spelled out "Fuck all editors" and "So long, Bulletin."*

Harwood's pseudonymous poems are daring inasmuch as they explore feelings that women, mothers in particular, have but are not supposed to have. As "Miriam Stone," Harwood wrote "Burning Sappho," in which the mother confesses: "Something like hatred forks between / my child and me."† In a poem written as Walter Lehmann, "In the Park," a woman whose children are bickering sees a former lover stroll by. She tells him that she likes to watch her kids "grow and thrive." But after he leaves, she rhymes bitterly: "They have eaten me alive."

According to Frances Lenado, the work of Gwen Harwood as Walter Lehmann exemplifies the "identity fluidity" that (she argues) marks great poets from Shakespeare and John Donne to Keats and Emily Dickinson. In Lenado's words, Harwood demonstrates that it is "liberating to shed her actual identity and write as another person entirely—someone she might want to be if only for the length of a poem. The poem's the thing, not the poet or the group that the poet is taken as representing." Lenado argues also

---

* See William H. Wilde, Joy Hooton, and Barry Andrews, *The Oxford Companion to Australian Literature* (South Melbourne: Oxford University Press, 1994).

† See Jaya Savige, "Creation's Holiday: On Silence and Monsters in Australian Poetry," *Poetry*, https://www.poetryfoundation.org/poetrymagazine/articles/89027/creations-holiday-on-silence-and-monsters-in-australian-poetry.

that there can be "a transfer of identity" when author and translator (or author and heteronym) are of different sexes.[*]

The Walter Lehmann affair of 1961 continued the noble Australian hoax tradition established by the fabricators of the fabulous Ern Malley in 1944. It is added proof of the immense value, to a working writer, of pseudonyms and heteronyms. But to this observer the combination of Walter Lehmann and Gwen Harwood holds a particular appeal because my name is Lehman and my wife's maiden name is Harwood.

Walter Lehmann visited New York once when I was eleven or twelve. A widower, he was a sweet-natured man though capable of great pugnacity in his writing. When he found out that I was bereft—my beloved Dodgers had abandoned Brooklyn—he talked about tennis so enthusiastically, about such Aussies as Lew Hoad, Ken Rosewall, and an up-and-comer named Rod Laver, that I took up the game that spring and became an avid fan. I rooted for Laver, Borg, Sampras, Federer, each one a great champ. On my back recovering from surgery I got to watch Wimbledon and I have to say that John McEnroe, that onetime bigmouthed brat, is as astute and articulate a play-by-play man as any sport enjoys. Chris Evert is also excellent. Aside from the soon-to-retire Vin Scully, the best baseball announcers are the Mets' Gary Cohen supplemented by either Ron Darling or Keith Hernandez or both.

Some days when I lie on the couch under a quilt with a vacant or pensive look on my face Stacey asks me what I am thinking of. And half the time it's something like: Who will be playing first for the Mets this season? But I am also entertaining the idea of digging in the family archives for the acrostics Walter Lehmann was known to have written in Sydney and Melbourne in the 1960s.

---

[*] Frances Lenado, "Gender Fluidity and the Use of Heteronyms," *Contemporary Literature in Translation* (Spring 2016): 68–96.

91

Rowing in Eden

In Europe as a young man I was acutely aware of being alone. This is not a complaint. On the contrary, I think of that lonesomeness tenderly. I wrote stories in which the nameless hero is referred to as "the American." Certain melodies haunted me like a Stanley Kubrick soundtrack. In my mind as I walked in Paris, I heard *An American in Paris* and sometimes Luciano Berio's *Sinfonia*; at the Montparnasse-Bienvenue train station, the opening number in *Cabaret*; at the airport, Dionne Warwick, "Always Something There to Remind Me." At my father's funeral, Beethoven's Ninth, fourth movement. On the London underground, the Rolling Stones, "Play with Fire." The passengers' conversations I heard and failed to understand on the picturesque Nation to Étoile line on the Paris Métro were as romantically sublime as the Eiffel Tower observed twice a day, blue in the morning, gold in the evening. The people could have been talking about a missed doctor's appointment, a business reversal, or a bad boss, it didn't matter. The French language itself was as sexy as the goodbye kiss in a Claude Chabrol thriller about a murderous butcher who loves his wife "à la folie." I read a lot in cafés. It was in a café that Camus summed up modern man as someone who fornicated and read the papers. "After that, the subject will be, if I may put it this way, spent."*

---

* *"Si j'ose dire, épuisé."* In French the word *épuisé* means both exhaustion in the casual sense and the specific exhaustion that follows male ejaculation.

92

I Remember Mama

In August 2001, Stacey and I went to Copenhagen to take part in a conference centering on American poetry today. Lyn Hejinian, Anne Carson, Ron Padgett, Rosmarie and Keith Waldrop, Mark Bibbins, Juliana Spahr, and Charles Bernstein were among the other participants. Charles and Susan brought their son Felix with them. We sat at a harbor café watching the boats. My job was to deliver a lecture on the New York School on Wednesday at the modern museum and to read my poems Friday. I never got to do the latter, because of emergency phone calls from the States. My mother had to be hospitalized and my sisters had summoned me to handle the situation. So we changed our tickets, flew back to New York on Thursday and down to Miami the next day. In Miami I authorized the operation and my mother pulled through.

In her hospital room the young doctor visited and told her cheerfully that the prognosis was excellent. Then he said, "May I borrow your son for a few minutes?" She said, "Sure." I thought: Now the truth comes out.

"Come with me," he said. He walked briskly down the corridor and I rushed to keep pace. "In here," he said, opening the door to a nondescript conference room. "Take a seat."

Then he pulled some papers from the inside breast pocket of his sport jacket. He said, "I've been writing poetry, and I wonder whether you could read these pieces and give me an opinion." I was relieved, even more so when, on reading the pages, I saw some skillful lines that I could praise. I recommended that he take a writing course with Denise Duhamel at FIU, and I had Scribner send him the year's *Best American Poetry*. "You have a wonderful son," he told my mother.

If I ever told my mother that I was too frightened to do something, she would slap me around and say, "Don't give me that. You can do it."

From this woman who spoke English with a foreign accent and never went to college I got better career advice, smarter tips on romance and relationships, than from any professional counselor or therapist. Once when she was visiting me in Ithaca, staying in the extra room on Valentine Place, she took a phone call when I was out for the afternoon. I returned the call later that evening. My friend, I forget who it was, a very nice person, asked me who had taken the message. "Was she, like, your maid?"

I learned how to manage investments because my mother, from the time I was thirty, entrusted me to manage her limited funds and prepare her taxes. She lived frugally and took few vacations, and we invested wisely in blue-chip growth stocks.

All my friends adored my mother. She had a natural joie de vivre, and nobody could make better *Schnitzel mit Kartoffel und Gurkensalat*.

When my mother was eighty-eight, we bought her a first-class ticket so she could fly in comfort from Miami to Washington and attend the White House reception for the authors taking part in the National Book Festival. When the flight attendant offered to take her coat, my mother reacted as though the uniformed woman was going to confiscate or steal the coat. "No," she said. "It's mine. I paid for it." But my mother liked telling such a joke on herself. And at breakfast with Stacey she recited lines by Goethe, Schiller, and Heine that she had learned by heart as a schoolgirl.

In her last years, I would phone my mother every day during Chanukah and light the candles and sing the prayers with her over the phone.

She died on Mother's Day, May 10, 2009.

93

No Regrets

"No Regrets": great song as the young Billie Holiday did it in the 1930s and I heard it forty years later. No regrets, and no use complaining.

Still, I could kick myself for not taking Philosophy 101 with Arthur Danto and the "sequence courses" in eighteenth-century and Victorian literature.

I wish I had taken a second year of German and an extra semester or two of French conversation.

No question I should have spent the summer after junior year in Paris, as Paul Starr did. Both of us had received summer travel stipends. I picked Oxford, which had its pleasures though it was futile to try recapturing the joys of the previous summer spent in that enchanted place.

But I have no real regrets.

I don't regret my PhD but I almost do.

I regret losing my temper in 1969, 1973, 1980, 1989, etc.

I regret it that in 1971 a barmaid at Cambridge's Baron of Beef pub lost her job because I flirted with her. In my room she cried but I could do nothing to help her.

Do I regret dating X or breaking up with Y or being hurt and causing pain?

No, but I regret not making a pass at M, A, R, N, S, E, P, T, and B when I could tell they wanted me to do so.

I don't regret sleeping in the same bed with T, P, N, G, and J though we were chaste and kissed but didn't touch.

Do I regret the time I wasted when I had time to waste? I do not.

Do I regret leaving the dorm and living with my parents sophomore year? I do not.

I don't regret any romantic relationships except maybe two of them.

Nor do I regret the summer of 1973 at the art colony in Cummington, Massachusetts, where William Cullen Bryant was born. It was a democratic place and the people weren't getting any work done, which they blamed on lunch, so at one of the weekly meetings that drove me nuts, they eliminated lunch, which totally pissed off the chef, who felt they were dissing him, so he quit. I slept too late for breakfast and the do-it-yourself lunches consisted of unappetizing peanut butter and jelly sandwiches so I shed ten pounds and went skinny-dipping with Tom and Kate and Tom's sister when I wasn't reading Jane Austen and Delmore Schwartz or walking in the woods and the nearby graveyard. Ron drove up for a visit with Cathy. I met Adele Gladstone who made a black-and-white drawing of me that I have framed in Ithaca. She and I discovered Beethoven's Violin Concerto in D major, Opus 61. I asked Nana Bennett whether she thought a certain book was good and this lovely, charming Sarah Lawrence graduate thought about it and said, "Finally, no," which I used to kick off a poem dedicated to her titled "The Impulse to Say Yes." I wonder where they are today, these wonderful girls. When I came back to New York that August, I weighed 149 pounds, my lowest since college, and I splurged on a beautiful blue trench coat at Paul Stuart.

I regret my lack of confidence when I started at Newsweek—
I wish I had been more relaxed, happy-go-lucky, punning away,
having a good time. I had not wanted so badly to succeed at some-
thing since Columbia.

Also, I should have visited Fürth, the small town in Bavaria
where my father grew up.

There are two other things I regret but they will go unnamed
here not because they are so shameful but because I believe that
mysteries are sacred.

I do not regret the year I gave in to anxiety and fear. I was love-
sick, which was even worse than homesick. But I had Baudelaire
and Poe to comfort me. It was the year Nixon resigned, and Mau-
rice Girodias published a book called *President Kissinger*, and twice
a week I had to figure out how to teach freshman English at Co-
lumbia. Only after you do it do you realize that no one has taught
you how to do it, in which sense teaching resembles journalism
and nearly every other activity worth doing.

There was a night when I, drunk, left forty bucks on a sixty-dollar
tab and Stacey said it didn't matter because you never regret over-
tipping, and she was right. I have never regretted over-tipping.

I regret gaining ten pounds when I stopped smoking. But I took
them off playing tennis and swimming.

I regret losing some of my pocket notebooks and hope a few
may still turn up.

And I regret not shaving off my mustache before I finally did it
in 1978, in Ashokan.

Why did I buy shares in that solar energy startup in 1981?

Why did I waste a summer afternoon in 1976 playing golf
(badly) at Hamilton College? I don't know, but I don't regret the
swimming pool in Vence on a summer evening when everyone was
twenty-eight or twenty-nine.

I regret using semicolons in my prose when I started out.

And I regret giving a bad review to certain books of poetry in 1972.

But these (except for the mustache and the failure to visit Fürth) are minor things.

I have no real regrets.

Kierkegaard says, "Marry or don't marry—you'll regret it either way," which is profound, though I am married and I don't regret it.

Nor do I regret the nights we spent listening to Edith Piaf sing *"Je ne regrette rien."*

94

If I Could

If I could undo the damage I did,
I would: the cars I crashed,
the jaws I broke,
the ants I crushed with my bootsoles,
the plates I smashed, the people
in the car I crashed, the man
who died because I, as governor,
refused to commute his sentence,
the cop who fell to his death because
I had vertigo and couldn't save him,
the children who died because I sold
tainted penicillin on the black market,
the bat I beat to death with a broom,
the bruises, the scars, the arm in a sling,
the broken nose, the busted marriage.

95

The Scar

The injury left a lasting scar
from belly button to groin but
things said or done, or things I didn't say or do,
weigh me down, and not a day
but something is recalled,
my conscience or my vanity appalled.
So I quoted Yeats without knowing it,
vacillating from the worst hour of the night
to a day of little music and loud noise
when I took my lanky frame for a walk
down University Place, heading for the Knickerbocker,
and Wordsworth's line came into my head,
"Even such a happy Child of earth am I,"
though "God" had replaced "earth" in my mind

96

The Secret

I split open a green Calimyrna fig and saw the secret of the universe.

To be in a hotel room with you when one of us knows the secret and whispers it in the other one's ear is to give in to temptation and there is joy in the afternoon.

Get old. Feel generous. Take a breath of good clean country air. Water the plants. Prune the hedges. You have learned the secret.

She asked him: "Why did you sign your name in pencil?"

He answered: "So you can erase it."

Do not keep the secret to yourself. But know that you will divide it in half the moment you share it with someone else.

Drunk he tried to act sober, but she wasn't having any of it. When he collapsed she had to undress him and move his dead weight into the bed. Nevertheless she forgave him, because she was in on the secret.

97

Like a Hurricane

I said health was like peace—something we take for granted until and unless we're at war. The doctor nodded, but his simile beat mine. "The medical establishment treating cancer is like a vengeful spouse who makes your life so miserable you agree to leave her." Then he says, "Like a hurricane. She comes wet and wild and takes your house when she goes."

At long last: The correct diagnosis of the gastrointestinal woes that have plagued me ever since the surgery has been revealed. I have celiac, for which the only cure is strict adherence to a gluten-free diet—and at the moment nothing in New York is more fashionable. (Tennis great Novak Djokovic is on a gluten-free diet.) I have had ten months of misery. One test after another has failed to diagnose the problem. I have been treated for an evil condition called Cdiff and other things, but there were false positives and other mishaps and only now do I undergo the endoscopy that will confirm what the blood test indicated.

"You have a textbook case of celiac," the doctor says.

"So what do I do?"

"You give up wheat and rye and beer and bread and pastry and cereal and other things you don't care about—but eat all the natural produce you want, and in no time you'll start to feel better."

Gluten is the culprit. Glory be to God.

Now what other part of my body is crumbling? My back. My lower back, on the right side of my body. No cure but massage therapy and swimming will help. The massage therapist says, "The center of tension is your glute." There's that word again.

98

In the Eyes of the Beholder

The urologist held a test tube of clear yellow liquid up to the light and smiled broadly.

I feel better. I can hardly believe it. Even the neuropathy and skin ailments are better. They tell me I've always had celiac, only I was able to "manage" it until the chemotherapy and surgery. And it is amazing the difference the diet makes. No beer, no baked goods, no wheat or barley. And no dairy. It doesn't seem a major sacrifice considering how much better I am feeling and functioning.

My scan is clean: no cancer.

Today the sun is shining brilliantly and the sky is full of fluffy white cumulus clouds. Outside my window the Japanese lilac looks lovely and the pots of verbena, Angelonia, geraniums, and petunias are thriving.

Yesterday Stacey and I met a sixteen-year-old girl who has her learner's permit and has her eye on an SUV. She was born on June third. "I'm a Gemini, too," I said. She said, "Who's your twin?" And I wondered and still do. My working assumption all along is that the twin brothers were internalized in me—that I am like a common stock that has undergone multiple stock splits over the years. Or maybe I am the liaison between my father and my son, both of them left-handed men named Joe. But now the question took me by surprise and I thought about my penchant for fast friendships. My bosom buddies, best pals, all of them named Eric except for Dennis, Joel, Bill, Pete, Rob, Larry, Jamie, Lew, Steve, Ron, Jim, another Joel, Glen, Tom, Mark. But perhaps the twin is of the opposite sex, in which case my twin is Stacey, who reminds me that she is a Leo with Gemini rising—the exact inversion of my birth and rising signs.

On the radio, Sinatra is singing "Walking in the Sunshine (of Your Love)" followed by Michael Bublé's "Sway." Maybe the best male vocalist out there today, Bublé has canceled his tour upon news that his son Noah has been diagnosed with liver cancer.

Now they're playing Sinatra's 1957 Seattle concert. Magnificent singing, but then he tells jokes. Bad ones. Mrs. Lincoln to Abe: "I don't care what you say, we're going to the theater tonight— it took me six weeks to get those tickets." And: "There's been an atomic explosion and there's only one man left and he's lonesome so he jumps off a tall building and as he falls he hears a phone ringing on the seventeenth floor." But then he sings "Violets for Your Furs," with "My Funny Valentine" on tap, and all is forgiven.

99

Champagne Cocktails

Ah, July. Food tastes like itself. The pure produce of America is fresh, a bounty of berries, cherries, a cantaloupe with port wine in the hollow, and I've renewed my taste for cocktails, the standard martini and Manhattan, the historic Lucien Gaudin (gin, Campari, dry vermouth, Cointreau), and the complicated concoctions that a good bartender will come up with. For every summer of my adult life since 1990 there is a drink. One summer it was the daiquiri; another year it was white peach sangria and bellinis. This summer I have dedicated to champagne cocktails and the sparkling white wines of the Finger Lakes, such as Chateau Frank Brut, Dr. Konstantin Frank, méthode champenoise, 2009. As far as I'm concerned, "champagne cocktails" can give "summer afternoon" a run for the money as the sweetest two-word phrase in the language.

For the first time in three years I don't wake up feeling sick, dreading the day. I have color in my face, and though I'm twenty-five pounds lighter than I should be, that's just as well. The strength is returning to my arms, my legs. I feel my shoulders expand with every stroke when I swim. My legs hurt the next morning but it's a good feeling—muscles unused are springing back to life.

It is not as though I have no pain. Every day there is pain. My feet hurt. When I stand too fast I get dizzy; I am prone to vertigo, and if I eat the wrong thing, my body rebels at three or four in the morning. My skin itches like hell where the prosthesis fits, and then there is the worry that it will fail, as has happened, embarrassingly. But this is pain I can live with.

Today a woman interviewed Stacey and me for an oral history project about cancer patients and their "caretakers."

What was the worst thing that happened?
How did you get through it?
Did you ever imagine dying as a relief from the misery and pain?
What did you learn from this experience?
When you looked over your life, what didn't you like seeing?
What will be different from now on?
When did you stop thinking that you might die?

The questions are impossible to answer except for the last (never: you never stop remembering that you will die).

100

In the Swim

I've been saying it all along with bravado but today I mean it: I am going to live. Like all cancer patients, I know that this is just a reprieve, temporary and subject to sudden reversal at any time. We are like middleweights obliged to defend our championship belts every three months. But it feels so good in the heat of July to stand up straight and tall and walk across the garden like a man who is going to live.

The sun warmed my body after I swam for twenty-five minutes in a blue pool some fifteen feet deep. I used to like diving into the pool. Can't do that anymore. Today I love feeling my shoulders my arms my belly my legs as I swim vigorously in the sun. May it always be summer.

The cancer research center gets in touch. In one hundred words or less, what five things would you tell someone who is diagnosed with bladder cancer?

- Always bring a trusted companion to every medical appointment. You will not be able to remember everything you hear.
- Confirm all appointments. No matter how well run the hospital is, there are always emergencies, scheduling errors, or failures of communication. We drove 250 miles for a procedure only to be told that it had been canceled three days earlier.

- Plan on winning the battle, but prepare your mind for the worst.
- Even on bad days, there are pleasant hours.
- You can do it. You can take it. It is amazing how much pain the body can withstand.

I want to keep it positive, though I know that there will be days, especially in the cold weather months, when one or another souvenir of my ordeal will flare up and make it difficult to get out of bed in the morning. Depression: big time. But as Porgy says in the Gershwin song, "No use complaining." Got my gal, got my Lord, got my song.

Even on days when I ache, I take pleasure in walking up or down a flight of stairs knowing there may come a time when I will no longer be able to do so—and recalling how, as a little kid, I learned to climb one step at a time, and then found I could manage it with one foot per stair rather than two. My family lived on the third floor and some days I would walk up the stairs to the fourth floor just for the pleasure of walking up and down an extra flight of stairs.

Two cups of coffee, and I'm in a state of exalted nervousness. On the radio: Tommy Dorsey, "Boogie Woogie" (1943). Chick Webb. "Blue Moon." Bea Wain. Lee Wiley, "Looking at You." Duke Ellington, "In a Sentimental Mood." And Ella and Louis are putting all their eggs in one basket. "I'm betting everything I've got on you." May the music of the 1940s last forever.

Odd notes: Cancer is the Alien in the Sigourney Weaver horror movie franchise. The 1960s advertisement for Tareyton cigarettes showed a man or a woman with a black eye and a tagline in defiance of correct grammar: "Us Tareyton smokers would rather fight than switch." I didn't think of it at the time but it now seems obvious that the sentence means "I'd rather get cancer than stop smoking." The shiner, too, is significant. It is like Moshe Dayan's eye patch, very virile. That's why Stan, the art director in *Mad Men*, has a poster of Dayan on his bedroom wall.

My old idea: cigarette brands named after all the astrological signs (Gemini, Leo, Virgo, Scorpio, Capricorn, Aries et al.) except for Cancer.

I can make that joke. I'm in excellent health.

—*November 2013–July 2016*